Living with Death without God

stories and solace for non-religious mortals

Valerie Jack

Finite Books

Published in 2023 by Finite Books

ISBN: 978-1-7393339-0-4

Cover image: 'Ash Leaves under Blue Sky II' used with kind permission from the artist, Julian Perry. (www.julianperry.info)

The wise words of Snoopy in conversation with Charlie Brown have been used by kind permission from Peanuts Worldwide, LLC. The author gratefully acknowledges the use of the following texts: *Somewhere Towards the End,* Copyright © Diana Athill 2009, Granta Books; *Alive, Alive Oh!,* Copyright © Diana Athill 2015, Granta Books; *The Denial of Death,* Copyright © Ernest Becker 2011, Souvenir Press; *Raising Freethinkers,* Copyright © Dale McGowan 2009, Thomas Nelson, reproduced by permission of the author; 'A Scattering' by Christopher Reid, published by Arete Books, 2009, Copyright © Christopher Reid, reproduced by permission of the author c/o Rogers, Coleridge & White Ltd., 20 Powis Mews, London W11 1JN. Extracts from the following texts have been reproduced with permission of The Licensor through PLSclear: *Every Third Thought,* Copyright © Robert McCrum 2017, Picador, reproduced by permission of Pan Macmillan; *The Meaning of Things,* Copyright © A.C. Grayling 2002, Phoenix, reproduced by permission of Orion Publishing Group Limited; *Non-Religious Pastoral Care,* Copyright © David Savage 2018, Routledge, reproduced by permission of Taylor & Francis Group; *Portraits from Memory and Other Essays,* Copyright © Bertrand Russell 2020, Routledge, reproduced by permission of Taylor & Francis Group; *What is Post-Traumatic Growth?,* Copyright © Miriam Akhtar 2017, Watkins, reproduced by permission of Watkins Media Limited; *Staring at the Sun,* Copyright © Irvin Yalom 2020, Piatkus, reproduced by permission of Little Brown Book Group Limited; *The Gift of Therapy,* Copyright © Irvin Yalom 2010, Piatkus, reproduced by permission of Little Brown Book Group Limited; *The Wiley Blackwell Handbook of Humanism,* Copyright © Andrew Copson and A.C. Grayling 2015, reproduced by permission of John Wiley & Sons Limited.

CONTENTS

1   **Beginning at the End**   1

2   **Where We Come from and Where We Go from Here:** *my story, i*   4

3   **Jane** *and non-religious pastoral support, i*   7

4   **John**: *here and now, reality is sufficient*   13

5   **Linda**: *a role model for facing death*   20

6   **Not Knowing How**: *my story, ii*   26

7   **A Fear Brewed in The Guts** *and how secular philosophy may or may not help*   28

8   **Matthew**: *looking inward and reaching outward*   33

9   **On Joining Song**: *secular community and connection*   42

10   **Someone at Your Bedside**: *non-religious pastoral support, ii*   51

11   **Louisa**: *the fact of happiness still stands*   54

12   **Margaret** *and non-religious funerals*   61

13   **Mariam and Zaheer**: *when the funeral doesn't fit*   65

14   **Arthur**: *in our life there is a single colour*   68

15   **Bob** *and his search for meaning in a living place*   76

16   **An Ongoing Search for Meaning**   87

17   **Roger** *and the treasure chest of memories*   90

18   **An Ending When We'd Just Begun**: *my story, iii*   93

19   **Claire** *and secular support when a baby dies*   97

20   **Kim**: *when we look at the stars, we'll think of her*   100

21	**11:11 and Other Moments in Time**: *my story, iv*	109
22	**Alison**: *just because you haven't seen a unicorn…*	112
23	**In Our Hearts and in The World**	121
24	**Sophie**: *going through the big stuff young*	125
25	**Alan:** *the expert widower*	131
26	**The Nature Prescription**	136
27	**Diana and Bridget** *and good that comes from loss*	138
28	**There But For…**: *my story, v*	143
29	**Tristan**: *how to live knowing time's not endless*	146
30	**Before I Die**…*and the death awareness movement*	154
31	**Flipping the Story**: *the days on which we live*	157
32	**Paul and Jenny**: *life is one big learning curve*	160
33	**Phil**: *speaking for those who want to live and die with dignity*	170
34	**Only When it Feels Like a Gift**: *religious influence in the assisted dying debate*	181
35	**Nathan and Bernard**: *a trip to Switzerland*	185
36	**CA125**: *my story, vi*	190
37	**Ruth**: *choosing how to live with a killer in the room*	192
38	**Strange Times**: *on regaining balance when the earth shifts*	207
39	**Jeffrey** *and being part of something bigger than ourselves*	213
40	**Last Words**	222

This is a work of non-fiction, researched and written over a period of six years. Many of the names have been changed to protect the privacy of those who shared their stories.

1

BEGINNING AT THE END

Are you ok with the fact you'll die and so will everyone you love? I never have been.

Religion promises a happy ending for believers; for millennia, many have turned to the stories of religion to cope with the hard fact of mortality. Some take comfort, believing in a loving watchful God; find meaning, believing human lives unfold according to His plan. When a loved one dies, some are consoled by the hope they'll one day be reunited in eternity and that when they close their own eyes for the last time, it won't really be the end.

Like more than half of the UK population, I have no religious faith. Yet being human, I still yearn for comfort, hope and meaning. This book has been my quest to discover what kind of happy ending may be possible for us non-believers.

I've been scared of death for as long as I remember. When I was around eight, I wrote a poem in which my entire family had died and I had to live in an orphanage that was all grey socks and damp walls. I didn't learn to drive as a teenager, thinking if I tried, I'd die in a car accident. About to turn 30, I resolved to take the wheel and live less fearfully. I took lessons and passed the test. Then, at 35, I decided to look at death head on. By that time I'd brushed against my own mortality and that of those I love most, and I'd experienced loss. But I felt ill-equipped to deal with those experiences and was frightened of the future. So, I set out to speak to people who are as expert in these matters as we humans ever can be – the ones who've lost those closest to them, or who are facing the prospect of their own, possibly imminent, death.

Between these pages, you'll meet people who know about darkness, yet still look for light and laughter. Bob finds life and fellowship at the natural burial ground that is his wife's last resting place. Kim's baby lived for only eight days yet left a lasting impact on her mother's heart and on the world. Matthew, who has prostate cancer, lives alone but learns to join song with others travelling a similar road. Ruth has a global pandemic to contend with on top of secondary cancer; while she can't choose her circumstances, she *can* choose to focus on all that remains possible. I weave personal experiences – my own and others'– with broader reflections about how we can help ourselves and each other through the toughest of times.

Every experience of grief, and every confrontation with personal mortality, is unique. No book could cover all possible circumstances of loss and illness, and all possible responses to those circumstances. But I have spoken to older and younger people; people with a close-knit family and others who look more to friends and community for mutual support through tough times; people who grew up in Christian, Jewish or Muslim households and others raised without religion; people who've struggled to reorient themselves following a loss of faith later in life and others who feel their secular beliefs have helped them weather adversity better than any religion could have. It has been a privilege to be entrusted with those most tender and personal parts of life that usually lie hidden. I've been allowed access to letters, diary entries and text messages; and have been invited to some of the places and events that feature in these stories. Each contributor offered up stitches towards a tapestry of human experience.

My hope is that if you are going through difficult experiences yourself, these stories may offer the comfort of companions as you travel your road. If you know people who are grieving, or who are nearing the end of their own lives, this book may enrich your understanding of how best to support non-religious people through tough times. Perhaps you are not, at this moment, in the eye of any storm of loss or illness but feel the time has come to begin addressing the questions this book asks. In the wake of our collective ambush by a global pandemic, many of us have been jolted into a heightened awareness of how precious and vulnerable our lives are. Recent research found the Covid-19 pandemic has encouraged more than half of us to think about our own mortality, with many of us now feeling more comfortable to talk about grief, and more compassionate towards others who are grieving. These last few years have prompted us to take stock. If you are asking yourself how best to live, given the fact of death, if you're looking for words to live with that feel hopeful, meaningful and true, then welcome – the stories between these pages are for you.

2

WHERE WE COME FROM AND WHERE WE GO FROM HERE

my story, i

When people ask why I've felt compelled to write about death, there isn't one big motivating experience I can point to. I think part of the answer lies beyond narrative reach, encoded in my above-averagely-anxious genes. But it also feels true to say that, growing up, no one handed me any map I could use to navigate the dark and difficult territories of life. With this book, I have been trying to find my way.

As a choirboy my father was pleased to earn two and six when he sang at weddings, and a whole five shillings for funerals. But when the time came for him to be confirmed in the Church of England, he refused. His life to that point, with parents who didn't show him love, had revealed no hand of God at work. When I told a friend my dad's philosophy on life, they checked they'd heard me right – 'to enjoy?' But no, my dad believes the purpose of life is 'to endure.' We're born, we die, and in between, try to go on with the things we're duty-bound to do.

At the C of E primary school I attended in the 80s, the 'daily act of collective worship,' still a legal requirement today for UK schools, was taken fairly seriously. We'd file into the hall, sit in cross-legged rows and be required to sing hymns of praise. I'd move my mouth to the Lord's Prayer

4

but not say the words. Though my dad never spoke about his atheism to me when I was young, I shared it. To me, Christianity was a far-fetched story I had no use for. But my dad's pessimistic philosophy of life being about gritting teeth until the road runs out wasn't useful to me either.

My mum was just three weeks old when her father suffered a fatal brain haemorrhage. For her mother, Lilian, it was devastating to become a widow at 44, with a small and - we think - unexpected baby to take care of, as well as a 14-year-old son and a business to run. Baby Mary lived with an aunt and uncle till she was two. Whenever teenaged Mary tried to ask her mother about her father, or about those first years after he died, Lilian would get too upset. Her generation had lived through two world wars; there'd been so much death and loss, and the tacit policy was not to talk about those things.

Lilian was a woman of faith who felt it natural that 'the days of our years are threescore years and ten.' At her 70th birthday, a gathering of the clans, she announced, 'That's it, I've had my lot,' and seemed at peace. Soon after, she suffered a major stroke. My mum took my eldest sister Eleanor to visit at the care home. She supported the baby in her mother's arms, as Lilian tried and failed to verbalise a response. Her death felt too soon for my mum, who, as a late-born baby, had reached just 28.

Losing her mother made my mum want to believe in some form of afterlife. Decades later, a spirit medium said her mother is with her in the flat where she lives alone, that when she is sitting on the sofa, her mother sits on the armchair. And that Lilian's spirit has been reunited with her husband, Llewellyn. These were consoling things for my mum to hear. Sometimes she feels her mother's presence at her shoulder, strongly enough it's as if she could turn around and see her. I don't begrudge my mum this comfort, but I've never been able to believe in supernatural happy endings myself.

My parents have had to find their way as best they could through dark and difficult territories; I've known their way can't be mine. With this book, I have been asking strangers for directions. I am an introvert, unsure how to be with people at the best of times. Setting out on this project, I was scared about approaching people living closely with death – of getting things wrong and making people in bad situations feel worse for speaking to me, of how the conversations I was seeking would make me feel. In the early days, I reassured myself that if I needed to, I could drop this book and do something else instead. I had that luxury of choice, to duck death for a while. Yet, curiosity and a desire to connect compelled me to stay with my questions and see where they took me.

I'm glad I did, because the people I've met and the stories they shared have helped me sketch out useful paths and landmarks on my map. They've shown me ways to live well in the face of illness, loss and fear; ways to live with death without God.

3

JANE

and non-religious pastoral support, i

One December morning in 2016, I set off nervously in the half-dark to drive to Leicester for the first conversation of this book. Jane Flint had been in post nearly a year, as the first non-religious pastoral carer employed by the NHS. I wanted to ask her about her work supporting staff, patients and their families through often very difficult experiences.

I'd done some background research. I knew that nearly half of us in the UK die in hospital; it is where very many of us will visit loved ones for the last time and live our own last days. When the NHS was established in 1948, it was intended to meet the needs of the whole person; Anglican chaplains were appointed to offer spiritual and emotional support to patients and their families. Many hospital chaplaincy teams have diversified in the last few decades, to better reflect the multi-faith communities they serve. However, until recently, non-religious patients and families have been left without appropriate pastoral support. The Non-Religious Pastoral Support Network (NRPSN) is beginning to address this gap in provision in UK hospitals and other institutions, through training non-religious pastoral carers.

Being non-religious may often not feel relevant to our relationships with others. We may be united in mutual support by any number of shared interests or circumstances – it could be walking, football, photography, or a diagnosis; beer, embroidery, books, or bereavement that brings a group of people together. There are times, though, when it may feel more pressing to be with someone who shares similar beliefs. In 2015, NHS England released guidelines which stated that 'people who do not hold a particular religious affiliation may still require pastoral support in times of crisis,' and that the non-religious should have equal access to such support. At critical moments, many of us would want the support of someone who sees the world as we do. A 2017 poll found that only 4% of non-religious people have ever used a chaplain, yet three quarters of us believe institutions which offer a support service from chaplains should also offer a dedicated non-religious pastoral support service. Furthermore, nearly half of non-religious people said that if they felt unhappy or concerned, they would be likely to seek support from a non-religious pastoral carer, were that support available. In January 2016, in response to the new NHS England guidelines, Leicester became the first hospital trust to create a paid post for a non-religious chaplain - Jane Flint. In the hospital cafeteria, Jane shared with me some experiences of her first year supporting patients, families and staff.

*

When she walks onto a ward and looks around, someone will make eye contact, so she'll go over. Many people, stuck in bed, will light up when she stops to talk. Then there are those who visibly back off. It's the ecclesiastical purple of the name badge, one woman told her; it's the word 'Chaplaincy' – even coming after 'Pastoral Carer.' She'd sometimes wear black, till someone took it for religious garb. Now she chooses colours with care, the blue-rimmed glasses, the magenta cardigan. When she did a presentation at the Secular Hall, one of the older guys took exception to the words she used referring to her role. She invited him to come up with something more appropriate, but it was paragraphs, you'd need a magnifying glass to read it on the badge. So she's 'Pastoral Carer, Chaplaincy.'

She started without a template. No 'This is what you're going to do,' more 'Oh, ok, you're here now!' The service she offers is so new that most people wouldn't know to ask for it. But a thousand new leaflets – 'Here for You, Support for People Who are Not Religious' – are gradually spreading the word. It was the same when the Trust first employed minority faith chaplains; it took a few years for word to get around. One of the first things is getting her post known amongst the medical staff. Some say, 'You're working in the chaplaincy but don't believe in God. I don't get it, what do you do then?' It's as if they think patients who aren't religious don't need anything or have beliefs at all. She wrote a load of polite emails to introduce herself and waited for replies. Of course, by then you're at the bottom of a 200-message pile.

Approaching her second year in-post, Jane was beginning to make headway, seeing a steady increase in people asking for the non-religious member of the chaplaincy. When you're vulnerable, and maybe scared, you want someone to be there, who can listen and not judge. Before the post started there were objections from a few colleagues, saying 'We already do that.' But the Head of Chaplaincy and others on the team believe in patient choice. If you're facing death and don't think you're heading somewhere else, you might not want someone next to you who thinks you're off to meet your maker and your mum. There's comfort in being with someone who has a roughly similar view of what's happening, in knowing, *ok, I'm not the only person in the world who thinks lights out, that's it.* Jane met a woman in her dying phase, only a brief chat as the nature of the woman's illness made it difficult for her to speak. Virtually the next day, she'd lost what little ability had been left, so it was never a discussion. It was going and sitting, with the patient knowing that here was someone with a similar worldview.

For the woman's brother, it was excruciating to sit in silence. So Jane asked 'Does your sister have any favourite books or poetry?' and he remembered she liked Robert Frost. Jane printed out a bunch of poems, which he then sat and read to her. When it comes to what brings comfort, there's no one size fits all. This woman is in a side room, the walls magnolia, bare. Jane would love to bring a poster, something to look at, if these walls will be the last this woman sees. When they first met, the woman motioned that she liked the colour of Jane's top, but the clue is not enough. Jane might bring something *she* likes, but which for this woman may be a torture in her last hours. The Christian chaplains have a box of little wooden crosses, rounded, smooth. A thing like that is nice to touch, to hold, but what can you give to someone who is not religious? There are conversations to be opened up and had there, you try to find out what might bring comfort to that person, but if you don't belong to some doctrine that has rules and rituals, there is nothing universal. All you can do is simply meet the person as an individual, try to find out what is comforting to *them*.

Thirty years or so ago she was in hospital herself, needing an operation. She recalls being taken through the admissions form:

'Ok, religion?'

'Well, none,' and they're moving to the next question, but she asks, 'What does that mean now I've said none?'

'Well if you were religious, you could see the chaplain if you wanted to talk to someone.'

'Who do *I* talk to then?'

'Sorry, there's no one.'

It was not particularly that she needed someone, but as a single parent of scared-stiff teenage kids, it would have been nice to know there was someone for them. And it got her wondering, what does that mean, when you're asked your religion and you answer none? She'd like to see the form changed to 'Religion or Belief,' because what the question tries to ask is what has meaning for this person, how can we support them?

For the most part what she does is ad hoc. She responds to what she finds. If they're able, she'll find a quiet room to go to, but many can't get out of bed to do that. It is difficult to hold a confidential conversation when you've got a patient either side. Still, you've come to be with them. You haven't come wanting to take their temperature or blood. Of course, some of the nurses are terrific listeners, but their focus has to be on physical care. You are the person who can take the time to sit. And they tell you they stole a bicycle when they were ten, or they always hated their mother, and you listen till they've said what's on their mind. Jane may see the person just that once, but before she goes she asks if they'd welcome another visit and if so, she makes a note. If that person's still in the next week, or is re-admitted, Jane will know here's someone for whom she's established some support, so that continues. When someone is dying, drifting in and out of consciousness, likely on a cocktail of drugs for pain control, when that person opens their eyes and sees she's still there, there's comfort in that for them. Sometimes Jane thinks of when her kids were small, the hours she'd hold their fingers as they fell asleep, so they'd know they weren't alone. She cannot guarantee she'll be there when somebody dies, but she can help the relatives to not feel guilty that they're human too and may need some rest. She can spend some time.

There was a gentleman she supported through his dying phase, five weeks or so, not every day, but whenever she was in that hospital she'd visit him. Afterwards, his daughter let her know how much it meant to him to talk to her, not having to go to the nth degree to explain himself. She'd brought interest to his afternoons, looked with him at the path he'd taken through life, helped him feel that it had been worthwhile.

When someone's reflecting on their life, as people tend to do when the end is in sight, they'll look at what they've done or haven't and try to see, *is there somewhere I have made a mark*? Whenever a patient talks that way, Jane remembers someone from her time working in the field of domestic abuse: a woman who left an abusive relationship after many previous failed attempts. Jane asked what had finally made the difference and this woman said how the times before when she'd been to Housing she had felt exposed and ashamed, standing right beside the large foyer window. But then one day instead of just speaking across the counter, the lady at the housing service took her to a private room to talk. It was seeing what respect looked like that made the difference. At the time, Jane thought to herself *that person who stepped out from behind the counter may never know the difference she made to another woman's life*: that being shown this simple human courtesy strengthened her to leave a man who would have killed her some day down the line. So, when a patient's hunting back through life and asking if they've made a mark, Jane tells them not to disregard the tiny things they may well not remember. Sometimes it's the act, the phrase that seems of no consequence which matters for another person. If you have never had your name in lights, written a book or invented something, your life still matters. Suppose one day she meets someone who's lived in total isolation like a hermit and has truly gone through life unnoticed? Well then, what she can offer is 'I'm noticing you right now and I'm listening to your story.' For patients to hear 'You're not invisible' makes a difference – she sees it in their faces.

Even a very early baby that doesn't survive has lived and made its mark. In the hospitals there will be a cot with a little chilled mattress, so that even in summer there's no rush to take the child from its parents. Mum and Dad can stay overnight in a double bed and have that time to say goodbye. For Christian parents, there's a Certificate of Christian Baptism to mark the life of their child, however brief. For non-religious parents the need is still there, but the language isn't fully formed. Non-religious couples sometimes ask for a blessing, not knowing what else to call it. Jane can put together words to mark that this small being lived and died, words she speaks aloud and then puts into their hands when the time comes to go home.

It isn't always non-religious families who ask for Jane. There was a church-going couple, who asked for her because they wanted to talk about things that might have gone against religious teachings. Jane's colleagues said, 'Of course we wouldn't judge, we're not like that.' But Jane understands that patients and families in crisis can't take the time to get to know staff personally. This couple wanted a clear space to think, without worrying about the reaction of the person they were talking to. They had to decide whether it was time to switch off life support. The couple were not talking, each hearing the other's silence as disagreement. After listening to them separately for a while, Jane was able to suggest, "Actually, you're both afraid, and wanting to protect each other by saying nothing. But you don't have the differences you think you do." Later they thanked her: they'd been in a stuck place, and she'd helped them to move out of it together.

Jane has a life outside these hospital buildings. The triumphs and disappointments of three grandchildren to absorb her. A dog to take through his agility paces. He's fast and the moves are complex; in that moment, there isn't room for other thoughts. But when a person's circle of existence has shrunk so that it's just a bed and whoever sits down next to it, Jane can be the one who sits awhile and listens. As she walks away their story ripples out.

*

I went to Jane with a long list of questions intended to elicit her insights on life, the dying process, the human condition, the universe... There was so much I wanted to better understand and she was the first person I had the chance to ask. Jane was good enough to sit talking with me three whole hours, before eventually flagging and suggesting we might wind things up. She'd given me a lot to think about; she'd got me started.

I had contacted Jane directly, but needed a larger pool of people to speak to. Humanists UK agreed to reach out to their membership with my request to speak to non-religious people who were over the age of 70 or had a life-limiting illness. I asked for interviewees willing to share their experiences and insights in relation to mortality and happiness, with the hope of offering guidance and comfort to others. I wasn't sure how much interest there would be, but the responses came in thick and fast. I felt both honoured that so many were willing to speak to me about such a sensitive subject, and a little overwhelmed as I set about triaging messages.

4

JOHN

here and now, reality is sufficient

John's initial email to me was self-deprecatingly jocular – he couldn't believe he could be of any interest, but 'if you are short of volunteers and are scraping the barrel you are welcome to get in touch.' When I responded to thank him and let him know that my initial focus was to meet those with a life-limiting illness, John told me he was living with the degenerative, untreatable condition, Multiple Systems Atrophy. He was glad I'd had a high level of response, but if I found myself back to the 'scrapings' I was welcome to call on him. Of course, I didn't consider John a 'scraping.' He was the first person to share with me his story of living with life-limiting illness.

*

As a geologist, John has long been fascinated by the five great extinctions – the asteroids, eruptions and ice sheets that have extinguished life. When the Yosemite Caldera blows – and it is now showing uplift – it will almost certainly presage a major extinction. To his wife, Sandra, John's calm interest in such things is strange and frightening. To John, these cycles of extinction and renewal are simply facts. And now it's time to face the fact of his own approaching extinction. His prognosis says he has a handful of years at best. He's 71, an age which many fellow baby boomers would be bold enough to think still youngish.

Religious members of his extended family assumed his diagnosis would somehow change his view of things. But no. Despite the faith his parents held dear and wanted to pass on, it seems to John a gene slipped through that told him *question everything, all the time.* It interests John that there could be a genetic basis for atheism, and for faith. Back in our cave days, humans had to be hyper aware of movements around them. That tickle on the leg could be a dangerous insect. That rustle in the branches could be a tiger readying to pounce. Equally, it could just be the wind, or a rotten branch falling. But if you wanted to stay alive, it was safer to assume the existence of some being that had the power to kill you. So, many of the ancestors who lived long enough to pass their genes on - eventually encoding 21st century human beings – would have been the ones who believed there was a tiger in the tree. Natural selection favours beliefs that have kept us safe, which may help explain why many still believe in the existence of higher beings who hold power over life and death. Somehow John's made it this far though without assuming there are tigers – or gods – ready to pounce down from above. And now? No god has given him this disease; no god will save him from it either.

John has always understood life's over in a blink of geological time. We have to make each day count. He has been the kind of guy who'd disappear up into the Cairn Gorms with a tiny tent in winter. Heading into retirement, he still felt physically indestructible – the odd cut or bash, yes, but never poorly. They moved to Devon and John got his day skipper's yacht licence. He crewed on a racing yacht owned by Sandra's cousin - that was a thrill! Then they moved back up to Bucks, wanting to be around for the grandkids while their parents worked.

John was deputy head of a big inner-city school for many years and has always been used to taking charge of situations. His diagnosis hasn't changed his worldview, but it has forced him to learn and re-learn the growing number of things he's not in charge of any more. He continued with some tutoring work until he reached 70, a year ago. His symptoms took out of his hands the decision to stop. If you're a natural scientist, your vocabulary needs to be extensive, but John began to mislay the words he needed. With the 17, 18-year-olds it was sort of ok. They'd say, 'It's alright John, you'll get there in a minute.' But the 15, 16-year-olds wouldn't have the patience or maturity for that. With MSA, swallowing is no longer automatic. Often, immersed in his work with a student, John would forget to swallow and suddenly, a great dollop of saliva would drop from his beard. Sometimes, with a GCSE student, he'd be monitoring their learning across the range of subjects, not just science. He might, for example, be reading a poem with a student, and since emotional regulation is impaired with MSA, he'd find himself weeping uncontrollably at the poet's words. John had always taken joy in helping students learn. There was something special about tutoring, because after several years of weekly visits to their home, you become somewhat part of the family. He was sad to have to give it up.

A degenerative illness is a process of continual loss. The work of adjustment is ongoing, unremitting. John sees it as a chance to show his grit. The obvious narrative is of decline, but you can do your darnedest to tell yourself a different story. A story that points to what there is still to live for.

At the first MSA Trust meeting John attended there was a representative from a firm that makes incontinence kit. John was thinking *no, one of the best cures for incontinence is muscle control in the abdominal and pelvic floor, it's called internal fitness.* There is acceptance, and then there's giving up. He didn't want to take the pads for leaks, the walking sticks, those goodies they were handing out. He stopped going to the meetings because he found them too defeatist. And yet, some of the people there were very brave. If he's really honest with himself, he feels in limbo, in a forgotten place, because no effective treatments have been established for MSA. But then again he's *not* in limbo because he's busy within the framework of what he's got. Now is the time to hit the gym, eat loads of fruit and veg, get out in the woods each day with Gizmo Dog. You scrap with the disease, say *come out here where I can see you!* Is he winning? No, but he'll give ground grudgingly. He takes a certain delight in not letting the thing take over.

What did it feel like when he sold his motorbike because he could no longer pick it up? Bit of a pisser for a while there to be honest. Now he rides his bicycle, and strangely he can ride better than walk. When he gets his feet up off the ground, they're not a problem, because he's balancing with eyes and ears. Could he skipper a yacht now? No, he couldn't begin to do that, he'd drown fairly quickly. Could he get up a cliff face on the end of a rope? No. So how does he deal with that? He deals with it. You're left with whatever you're left with. Reality is sufficient, though it's a smaller sufficiency over time. Sandra still talks about getting on one of the long trails again, Offa's Dyke or something. *Don't talk, San.* But was he any happier walking Offa's Dyke than he was this morning up amongst the crocuses with Gizmo? Truly, no. You have to think *aren't I lucky?* Walking the dog in the woods is one of his daily delights. Always he works to focus on a can-do situation. And there are new things in his life now that he has retired fully. He is growing his involvement with the U3A, finding which groups are a fit for him. So far, he's enjoying the art, psychology and current affairs groups; enjoying conversation with people who are broadly on his wavelength, but who also hold some quite diverse views. Here and now, reality is sufficient.

The other evening, he was sitting with his legs up on the pouffe.

Sandra asked him 'Has the acupuncture eased your feet?'

'It offends me as a scientist, because I can't explain it, but yeah, look, I can wiggle my big toe.'

Their daughter Chloe had just popped in and suddenly got very upset to hear them chat this way. She *knows* what's wrong, she's read the paperwork, but sneakily wants it not to be the case. John tends not to go on about the realities of his illness because they – his wife, his daughter and his grandchildren – are dealing with their own grief at gradually losing him. Chloe hadn't realised her dad had already lost so much feeling and movement. It was hard for her to see him have to manually lift his legs to cross them round the other way. It was hard for John not to be able to take away his daughter's sadness. John thinks we don't really have anything to offer each other apart from the listening ear and the giving of time. He tries to remember that very often, those things are enough.

It's difficult at times, not to feel useless. He can't get up ladders any more, can't bring the breakfast tray down from the bedroom, because he can't rely on hitting the top step right. Instead of being an equal partner, moving smoothly in the roles of nearly half a century of marriage, he will be more and more dependent on Sandra, and that is very difficult to contemplate. To deal with what *is*, is the thing, and that means not too much of past or future. He can deal with all the things of now, as and when they come along. Occasionally, he will fetch down that hypothetical box marked 'Future,' open the lid and say *ok, let's take a look at Sandra as she almost certainly will be, Sandra without John.* How will she manage all the things that have always been his tasks? Because she's daft as a brush. Well no, she's very bright and competent. But he wants to leave things in the best possible order for her. So he'll take a peek inside that box when necessary. And he does ask himself – because they've been married 49 years – what sort of nick he'll be in when they reach the 50-year mark. As good as he can manage is the answer, but he doesn't look at that stuff too often or too long.

In fact, there's one new way John can be of use to other people. MSA is not well understood, so researchers are keen to find out all they can from those living with it. John has signed up for the national programme. He'll go periodically for interviews and tests over a three to five year period. For his first visit there'll be an interview that lasts five hours. *It had better be someone nice doing that!* Right now, they don't know how to combat MSA. Sometimes it's lonely, to feel no one can do anything for him, but it's some consolation to think he's helping with the research. And somewhere down the line maybe they'll develop drugs to help someone like him.

At present, John is still of use to his family as well. They are closely knit – in fact, John and Sandra's garden interconnects with Chloe and Marc's, so the grandkids are through here all the time. They get fed in the evenings when their parents are working. With Marc often working abroad, James can use John as his stand-in dad, to bounce ideas off; and Anna knows that Grandad is the soppiest thing on two legs, whom she can wheedle into anything. Yesterday, she asked, 'Grandad, whose face do I have?' Because she doesn't look like any family members she knows. John said, 'You've got my mother's face,' and took her upstairs to dig out a particular photograph. A photo of his mother aged 19, which way-back-when she put under his father's hospital pillow. That handsome young chap she took a shine to, after he came off his motorbike and she was part of the nursing team that saved his life. Nearly a century on, here stand John and his granddaughter Anna, looking at this sepia snap. And you could swear that was Anna looking back at you from 1920 something.

John's mother, when elderly, would always play with his hands when she saw him. One day, John asked 'Why do you do that, Mum?' She said 'You've got your dad's hands. It's like your dad is here.' That was a comfort to her. And the actual reality is that genetically, John's hands are almost exactly the same as his dad's. So he still exists. It's the bottom line: your family are you. Thomas Hardy wrote about the 'family face,' that lives on, leaping over oblivion, far beyond the reach of a single human span. He called that inheritance 'the eternal thing in man.' So, John has a future – James and Anna are 25% him. Can he recognise that 25%? Absolutely, yes!

And it feels good to know he's played a part in teaching them to see things as they are. The vicar, who lives next door, has known James and Anna since they were little and regards John's influence on them very negatively. What he doesn't realise is that John's never tried to influence them in any shape or form, other than that he talks to them about reality, and never about things that aren't real. When you look at the next generation and the planet we're handing them, there cannot be the optimism John's generation felt back in the 60s. There are big issues to be faced, but John takes comfort from the fact that across a 40-year career as a teacher he had an impact – hopefully positive – on thousands; he has raised kids, and has a hand in raising grandkids, who think for themselves, and who are absolutely capable of facing the most difficult issues there are. And they will do it well. James and Anna's other grandma lives in a rambling, ghost story place and she was amazed that Anna was absolutely content to be left alone in that house, aged 13. Of course, Anna's response was, 'I've got a Great Dane that would kill anything that threatened me, I've got phones, a police station around the corner, what's to be frightened of?' Anna and James will often come from their home here to John and Sandra's through the gardens in the winter dark, without nerves of any kind. They know there's little chance of someone lurking, no tigers in the branches of the fruit trees. Then, of course, San's frightened of absolutely nothing, including John! If the two of them have had something to do with building grandkids who'll walk fearless through the dark, for John, that is sufficient.

*

When I let John know we'd covered all my questions, he asked, 'Have you got enough?' checking he'd been useful to me. He mentioned that Sandra may also be willing to speak to me at some point. I saw the teacher in him as he indicated with gestures how to reverse out of the awkward spot I'd got my car into on his drive. We waved goodbye.

I've never heard from John since. I emailed him a couple of days after we met, thanking him for what he'd shared with me, and suggesting that perhaps we could speak again in a few months. When I didn't hear from him, I looked back at my message, which now looked crassly worded, saying I'd be interested in getting 'an update on your situation.' What 'update' can there be about the 'situation' of living with a degenerative condition that is getting progressively worse? Listening back to the recording of our interview, I noticed that more and more as our conversation went on, John posed and then answered his own questions. It seemed a way for him to hold on to some control, to block me from asking questions that he didn't want to answer. At one point, though, I asked about his hopes and fears for the future.

'That my wife's ok,' he answered, 'and that I'm not too much of a burden. Now that's going to upset me, so at this moment in time, I'm putting it back in the box.'

'Ok,' I said.

'I opened it for you, but it has to go back in now.'

'Ok,' I said, and we continued the conversation in a different direction.

Looking back afterwards, the humorous way in which John had introduced himself as a 'scraping,' seemed to reveal a stark truth. On some level, John felt useless, and that depressed him. With his diagnosis, John felt a sharp disjunction from his former life of usefulness to the thousands of students he had taught, and to his wife of 49 years.

Later, I contacted John again. I let him know that his contribution was valuable to me, and that the image of his grandchildren walking fearless through the dark has stuck with me. I asked him whether he would like to read what I had written based on what he shared. I didn't hear back.

While he was telling me his story, John had remarked 'this is most unusual.' He wasn't used to talking in such detail about what it's like to live with MSA. He noted, 'I can talk to you because you're a stranger.' I know there can be value in speaking to someone who is at a distance, who, unlike close family members, isn't dealing with their own grief. Maybe our conversation was of some use to John. I am uneasy that John, unlike most of the other contributors, didn't read through what I wrote about him and give it his ok. But he had begun his first email to me, 'I have been asked to see if I can be of any help with your research.' He wanted to be helpful, and at no point withdrew the consent he gave for me to use his story, so I have become comfortable to include it. Whatever has transpired for John since I met him back in 2017, I hope he found ways to continue to feel useful to those closest to him, and that he took comfort from his contribution to research into effective treatments for MSA. I hope you've found value in John's story, too.

5

LINDA

a role model for facing death

When Linda was 10, her grandfather died. She has a clear memory of standing in her back garden very frightened, thinking about cancer and *when will I die?* She could never talk to her parents about much, and her brother and sisters had already left home. She told herself *I don't have to think about that until I'm at least 20*, which seemed very far off, and that helped a bit. When, at 14, her thoughts returned to death she decided, *you needn't think too much about that until you're 28*. Which was very old. She'd do these doubling sums so as not to have to think about dying all the time.

Of course, now she can't duck it any longer. At some point you have to come to some accommodation with the fact you're going to die and with what may or may not happen after death. Someone you love dies, you're getting older and become ill yourself... Now Linda is 72. When she got the leukaemia diagnosis, on top of her heart arrhythmia, she realised she needed to slow down, and so she hired a delightful lady to come and clean the house, who, when she knew about the diagnosis said,

'Ah! You must be terrified! Are you praying to God?'

'I don't believe in God.'

'You don't believe in God? Oh my God, my God, I've got to pray for you!'

Linda's older sister, Rose, too, was contacting her church friends saying 'Pray for Linda!' *So what then*, Linda thought, *your God is up there calculating how many people are praying for Linda? 250? Touch and go. Only 5? No chance!* Linda can't imagine any God that created this amazing universe worrying how many people are praying for Linda Wright because she's going through a rough patch.

She had a faith once. When Billy Graham came crusading in the 50s, packing out Wembley stadium and preaching hellfire, Linda's sister, Rose, was one of the thousands who answered his call to come on down and accept Jesus into their hearts. Rose became a member of the Baptist Church, and lonely eight-years-younger Linda tagged along. Theirs was a working-class home at a time when you accepted the wisdom of people in authority – the doctor was always right, as were the teacher and the minister. Linda's school report said 'Asks too many questions,' but she tried to go along with things and be a good Christian. As she reached her teens, she made lots of friends at church and it was quite a comfortable cocoon, with people speaking the same language, reinforcing the beliefs. But when those friends began to go off their own ways, to colleges or jobs elsewhere, somehow Linda's faith began to drain away. She couldn't help but notice that for all the assertions of love and charity, people in the church weren't always kind.

At 22, pregnant with her second child, Linda went into what looked like premature labour. She was partly dilated and had to spend a week in hospital. When they sent her home, the doctor said 'Just rest and try to hang on for a few more weeks.' It wasn't easy with a two-year-old to care for; Linda had to watch from the sofa while he played. For several years, she'd been hosting all the young people from church after the Sunday evening service; they'd come round for a cup of tea and chat. She contacted the minister to say 'I'm really sorry, I'm going to have to stop having people back,' and he wrote a very formal reply saying 'You've let everybody down.' Linda could have done with a bit of help herself but wasn't going to ask for it after that. She managed to hold on till 37 weeks and Sally turned out fine.

Soon after, though, Linda's father had a heart attack. She prayed and prayed he wouldn't die. When he came through it she was so relieved – *he's ok, he's not going to die!* she thought. And almost the same instant – *but yes he is, and so am I.* It was one of those snapshot moments. Three years later, her father was admitted to hospital in excruciating pain. It was cancer of the bone marrow and there was nothing they could do. Linda had just moved away for her husband, Andrew's job; every weekend during those months, they'd drive round the North Circular in an ancient car with two children and a dog to see her father. She'd stopped going to church, stopped praying. Her remaining trace of faith was too weak to prop her up.

Her sister, Rose, was still devout, and beside herself because she genuinely believed their father was going to burn in hell. He'd always said 'I can't believe this person Jesus died on the cross and then came back to life, I just can't do it.' Rose frantically tried to convert him in his final days, telling him to confess and let Jesus in his heart, and he'd be saying, 'Please, just drop it.' Linda thought *if you truly believe this man who liked a flutter on the horses, but put food on the table and lived the best he could – if you believe he'll go to hell because he hasn't spoken certain words, there's something wrong here.* And that was the end of faith for Linda.

Linda was 26 when her father died and it was a very great loss. He'd been the parent who had shown warmth and was a loving grandad too. He had a chair with very broad arms. When six-year-old Dale was struggling with his asthma, he'd sit with Grandad. Looking back, Linda thinks she was close to clinical depression after her father died. She felt remote from her children for a while. One time she and Dale were watching some film about a little robot who gets lost in space. Suddenly, he burst into tears and said, 'Do you think that's what's happened to Grandad?' Linda felt lost herself; Andrew was establishing himself in a new job and on the political scene of this new town and they were heading for divorce. After a while, she got to know a few people in the area, one of whom suggested she'd make a good counsellor.

At the time, Linda was thinking hard about relationships and how they work; the counselling training helped her do that, so that in turn she was able to help others look at what was and wasn't working in their lives. When people came to her with their issues and anxieties, including those around death, she'd have them look at what is good today. The more you churn over your fears, the more they poison daily living. In the end, however depressed or anxious you may be about it, we're all going to go – you and everyone you love. The here and now is what we've got, so that's where we must put our energy. It's about finding the things you want to put in place - the relationships you care about, the activities you love - that can add up to a satisfying life. Don't beat yourself up too much about the past, don't fret too much about the future – right now you're here and you're alive. What can you do to make that life a good one, now?

The fact that life can end in an instant was made very real for Linda when Andrew died during a game of squash. He was only 49. They were long-divorced by then. Dale and Sally were in their early twenties and his death devastated them. If you know someone is ill and there's no way back, you do anticipatory grieving, so that when the person dies there's a sadness but often also a degree of relief. Sudden death is *hard* for those left behind. They couldn't *believe* he was gone; it took a long time to shake the feeling he was out there somewhere – even though the three of them went to the hospital together to identify his body. Andrew and Linda shared a birthday and he was two years older, so that felt very close. She remembers clearly on her 50th birthday, the strange feeling of having outlived him. Now, of course, it's so long ago, and she often thinks of all he missed. He didn't see his children married. He didn't see his grandchildren. How precious that Linda has had that time, and that, though she knows well she's not time-rich, she's still here to be a part of the family's unfurling. They are a family who do talk about people who are gone. She's worked hard to make it easy for Dale and Sally to talk about their dad, and for their children to hear about the grandfather they never knew, who was an interesting character.

Linda believes belonging to a loving group of family and friends is really what carries you through the tough times. The book club she founded is the tightest group she's ever been in – a room of people who can say anything to one another. She's been married to Neil more than 30 years now; his kids and hers have given them seven grandchildren. Linda knows quite a few people who feel increasingly pointless as they get older but she doesn't feel that. She can still spend time with the people she loves in a way that is enjoyable for both sides. If you have grandchildren, you get terribly involved with babysitting for the first five years, then as soon as they start school, they begin to have their own diaries and it becomes increasingly difficult to get the family together. When they're teenagers, they want to be with their peer group and they're not so keen on family events. And then of course they're off; it's a sort of staircase up and out into the world where they establish their own identities. But there's a lot of Facebook and texting and when they come to visit they'll sit and have a proper talk. About each other's lives of course, and about the world in which we live now. The grandchildren, aged between 16 and 24, think about the problems of the world and how best to play their part in solving them. They've been raised in families that talk about how to make society more fair. Alexis, the youngest of them, is small in stature like her grandmother, but fierce, and Linda loves it when she says, 'Granny I want to be like you – I want to be feisty and stand up for what I believe in!' To be at the hub of this family is a wonderful place! To have a much-loved grandchild claim her as a role model feels like a successful life!

It's ten years now, since Linda's leukaemia diagnosis. She's reconciled to the fact she may not have long left, though she cannot say she's overjoyed. She can imagine getting to the point, though, where she'd be glad to go. With chronic lymphocytic leukaemia, they talk about indolent periods. Two years ago, Linda's white lymphocyte cells were steadily climbing, but then they levelled off. The disease is in a quiet period. It's there, making her vulnerable to infections, making her tired and giving her increasing joint pains, so there's a sense it's getting a stronger grip, but it's not so bad. Because she has a heart arrhythmia as well, she's on one of the new anti-coagulants to lower her risk of having a stroke. It makes her eyes dry and blood-shot, all the time they're itchy. Little things like that incrementally change your experience of yourself, your level of enjoyment in your own body.

Modern medicine is brilliant, it keeps you alive, but it has its side effects. A friend invited them to her 90th birthday, saying 'This is Penelope's last Hurrah!' 50 people came to the tennis club for an amazing lunch and an afternoon of dancing, singing, poetry. Penelope was still tapdancing with her great grandchildren when Linda and Neil went over to say thank you and goodbye. Penelope said 'I'll tell you what I'm going to do now. I'm going home and throwing *all* my medication away. I'm fed up with it! I've got to 90, and I've had a lovely time today.' Linda can imagine getting to a similar point and thinking *that's enough*. She wakes each morning and her eyes feel like they've got sand in them. She tells herself *this is probably the worst you're going to feel all day, hold on to that thought*. She gets up and gets on.

There are enough things in her life worth getting up for. The interest in portrait painting she had no time for while at work and raising kids has returned now that she is retired. In the local humanist group she's found people whose beliefs and values match her own; people who volunteer – at the library or in sustainable transport - who do the things needed to make a decent society and look after our planet. Because if there's no divinely-ordained justice in a world to come, that just leaves us and what we do or don't do here and now. Though Linda's energy levels are low these days, she still tries to be part of the causes she believes in: she'll retweet about the royals spending millions of taxpayers' money on refurbishing their private homes, while our public services lie in tatters; she'll voice her support for those speaking truth to power about the climate crisis.

Linda has written an Advance Statement, which her GP has seen. It says basically if she becomes ill to the point there's no way back, she'd prefer to be at home, unless that becomes too difficult or distressing for her family, in which case she'd like to go to a hospice. She doesn't want aggressive intervention. She'd like the kind of palliative care that will keep her comfortable and may involve just a little too much morphine at the end. Neil knows her wishes, as do Dale and Sally; she has faith their judgement will be sound. They'll have clarity so won't need to argue or to guess.

After her leukaemia diagnosis, Linda wrote a series of letters, expressing her beliefs and sentiments about the people she loves best. Every now and then she has a look at what she's written, because it's been ten years – life changes, people change. The six-year-old is sixteen now, and Linda wants the words to feel up to date. She's tried to get her philosophy on life into a little bundle: that truth is the basis of trust and trust is the basis of love and if you think of those three things and the relationship between them, you can work through most stuff. That no one person can solve all the problems of the world, you just try to play your own small part. You try to balance the macro with the micro, and as often as you can, you enjoy the warm and wonderful things of life.

She would like to be a role model for her loved ones on how to face the final stage of life. She's always tried to be honest with them about what's happening with her health. The letters are a way of saying you can face up to these things without going to pieces. When you get there, the mind tends towards a reconciliation with your own end. She doesn't think she'll be looking down over them, but they'll have something from her. She knows it can be steadying to have some words about you from a loved one who has died. So now Alexis is 16; it would be something complete, to know what kind of path her youngest grandchild is setting out on. Linda knows her time is limited – every time she has a closer brush she thinks *hmm…* She'd like to stick around until Alexis reaches 18, or even 21. It might not happen, but the trick is not to let that knowledge spoil today. Today she's still here, still standing. Today is good.

6

NOT KNOWING HOW

my story, ii

Mum holds her best friend's arm and they stagger to the front row. This is my first funeral. I am 27. I was never christened, never officially had godparents, but if I had done they'd have been Nancy and Peter. After the service, I want to tell Nancy how sorry I am; but I start crying, so she has to be the one to comfort me about the fact her husband has taken his own life. *I don't know how to do this stuff.*

A year later, during a routine polyp removal on a Friday afternoon, a surgeon perforates Mum's bowel. They try to fix it, but she goes into sepsis, delirious with pain and fever. They give her tramadol. She's left alone, the only patient on the ward that night. She sees goblins at the end of the bed with horrible disformed faces, bright green, with bloody teeth and bulbous eyes. They're coming for her. She rings the bell and a nurse sits with her for a quarter of an hour but then has to get on with other things. I'm 28, the age my mum was when she lost hers. This makes her think she's about to die. She sees a figure sweeping a river of blood.

I'm not there with her. I'm miles away, feeling worried and useless. As the youngest in the family, I'm not top of anyone's list of people to call on in a crisis. And I haven't yet learnt to drive a car. The next week, I take time off from my work as a teacher and go on the train to see my mum. I am only half a helper. Dad has to ferry me from the train station to the supermarket to buy food Mum thinks she might be able to manage, then to the hospital to spend time with her.

She is 64 and suddenly frail. It's a big achievement when she manages to shuffle on my arm to the end of the hospital corridor. Then it's back to bed, where I read to her, massage her feet and lower back. The story is she's on the mend. They had to remove a section of her bowel to stop the bleeding, and say she will be able to go home once she's mastered changing the stoma bag. After a few days, my sister takes the next shift with Mum. I head back to my life.

They haven't fixed her. She haemorrhages. The consultant asks my sister to stay on the ward over night because Mum is seriously unwell. They don't know how to stop the bleeding. The surgeon, the consultant and a third doctor stand at the end of her bed scratching their heads saying maybe they could try this one last thing with gel and mesh but if that doesn't work, they don't know what else…

Mum didn't die that night. She gradually got better and we were able to let relief replace our fears. During her long recuperation, a visit to the hairdresser was the last thing on Mum's mind. She allowed herself to go grey, and was pleasantly surprised to find in fact her new hair came in soft and white. She also reassessed relationships, allowing those in which she'd always been the one to make an effort, to fall by the wayside now. A close call with death can draw our focus to what is meaningful and true. But, when Linda told me what happened in her head after her father pulled through a heart attack, I felt a jolt of recognition. The relief – *he's not going to die!* – but on its heels the flash of fear – *yes he is and so am I*. I still had my mum, but one day she'd be gone and so would I. It still felt like a problem I had to somehow solve.

7

A FEAR BREWED IN THE GUTS

and how secular philosophy may or may not help

When I began this project, the happy ending promised by religion seemed in its way a perfect solution to death anxiety – just that I, along with many others, found the promises of religion entirely unbelievable. I was looking for some kind of equivalent solution for non-believers. From Linda's initial email, I knew she'd had a long career in psychology and counselling; she seemed a good person to go to for answers. I was trying not to bring too much of myself to interviews, wanting to leave the space for people's stories. But Linda had my number. I asked her about clients she'd had – 'If someone was non-religious and they were talking about mortality and death or dying, how could you reframe that in a positive way?' This was a rephrasing of something I'd already asked. Linda said 'I get the feeling this is a question very much on your own mind?'

Yes, it was, it is. Part of Linda's answer was to point out that it's a mistake to think religious people don't fear death. She said, 'My sister is profoundly religious and I can tell you, she's not relishing the idea of the trumpet sounding up there, she's terrified of going, so it's not making much difference to her.' I'd been reading around my subject area for a year before setting out to speak to people, and continued reading as the project went on. My reading and my conversations led me to realise the promise of an afterlife isn't such a neat solution to death anxiety as I had thought.

The relationship between religiosity and death anxiety is an inverted U. That is to say, the very religious at one end of the scale, and the convinced atheists at the other are the two groups who experience the lowest levels of death anxiety. It makes sense that feeling certain about what happens after death would reduce anxiety. Richard Dawkins, on his scale of belief and unbelief, puts strong theists (100% certain that God exists) at number 1, strong atheists (100% certain that there is no God), at number 7, and himself at 6.9. I would probably put myself around 6.0. Most of us sit not at either extreme in our beliefs, but somewhere in between, uncertain, and feeling the anxiety that comes with uncertainty.

Even a strong religious faith usually can't eliminate death anxiety entirely. Dale McGowan, writer and speaker on non-religious parenting, is often asked 'Without heaven, how will you make your kids okay with death?' The implication is that religion cures the fear of death, but McGowan notes 'I know many deeply religious people, all of whom work hard at delaying their demise. They look carefully before crossing the street. They watch what they eat, follow doctor's orders, shrink in terror when given a troubling diagnosis.' McGowan points out that 'fear of death is among our healthiest and most desirable fears. Natural selection put it there, after all, for good reason.' He asks us to imagine two early ancestors crossing the savannah: 'one has a genetically endowed fear of death, while the other is indifferent to it. A predator sprints their way. All other things being equal, which of these guys will survive to pass on his attitude toward death?'

Some non-religious people I spoke to, when asked about fear of death, told me it wasn't death itself they feared, but what came before it, the dying part. I'm not sure whether there are really people out there who have zero fear of death. I know I fear both dying and being dead. Me existing is all I have ever known. The thought of not existing fills me with inchoate, jittery dread. Secular philosophers, ancient and modern, have done their best to persuade readers that to feel as I do is an error.

As humanist philosopher Peter Cave observes, 'a conscious being finds it virtually impossible to imagine unconscious non-being. Merely by attempting to imagine such a thing, we cannot help but place ourselves in the picture.' We may imagine experiencing endless cold blackness, worms or other horrors. In what is now known as the 'symmetry argument,' Roman philosopher Lucretius attempts to guide us towards a more accurate understanding of non-being, suggesting that we 'look back at the eternity that passed before we were born, and mark how utterly it counts to us as nothing. This is a mirror that nature holds up to us, in which we may see the time that shall be after we are dead.' Lucretius reassures us that, just as our state of non-being pre-birth held no terror, neither should the state of non-being that awaits us post-death. The 19th century novelist Mark Twain, apparently convinced by this line of reasoning, wrote 'I do not fear death. I had been dead for billions and billions of years before I was born, and had not suffered the slightest inconvenience from it.' Some non-religious people may take comfort from A.C. Grayling's suggestion that, though we have no belief in an immortal soul, 'from the subjective perspective, we are immortal,' since 'our own deaths are no part of our personal experience: each of us experiences only life.'

I asked some of my interviewees whether they felt reassured by secular philosophers. Walter, 82, told me that the other day, he'd consulted the life expectancy calculator on the Office for National Statistics website. Based on his age and sex, the calculator told him he could expect to live to 86. Disappointed with this verdict, Walter sought a second opinion from a calculator that allowed him to input additional information – that no close relatives had died of heart disease at a young age, that he exercises and doesn't smoke. He was able to get the number up to 93 and was happier with that. Walter doesn't want to die; he likes being alive, playing chess with his friends and tennis with his wife. It does help a little, though, to remember that his life is everything he has; when the moment of his death comes, he won't be there, that won't be him. Some years back, he heard the Ancient Greek philosopher Epicurus quoted at a funeral – 'Why should I fear death? If I am, then death is not. If death is, then I am not. Why should I fear that which can only exist when I do not?' That way of looking at death has stayed with Walter, and consoled him, ever since.

Some, like Walter, and like non-religious memoirist Diana Athill, have found consolation in philosophy. In her eighties, Athill reflected that death to her had never been frightening – for this she credited the French philosopher Michel Montaigne, whose advice she had taken to 'spend a short time every day thinking about death, thus getting used to its inevitability and coming to understand that something inevitable is natural and can't be too bad.' But something Athill noted a few pages on has stuck with me. She'd recently participated in a television programme designed by the photographer Rankin to help him overcome his fear of death. Athill wondered whether the programme served its purpose, speculating 'possibly not, because that fear is brewed in the guts, not in the mind.'

Reading philosophy didn't do much for the existential dread brewing in my gut. If it had, I suppose I wouldn't have needed to repeatedly ask Linda and others like her, in many different ways, what makes it ok that we're all going to die. It doesn't register in my gut that I don't need to fear being dead because I *won't* be dead, because I won't *be*. For her part, Linda told me how as a child and young woman she tried to push away the fears of death that threatened to overwhelm her. But at the point I met her, the thought of a final darkness falling no longer troubled her.

Being with Linda and hearing what she had to say helped me more than reading philosophy could. Linda has come to terms with death. Though she has dealt with and is dealing with difficult experiences of loss and illness, the main mood of our conversations was one of calm reflection. Aware she isn't time-rich, she has made her wishes known. She would prefer to die at home, unless this becomes too difficult or distressing for her family, in which case, she would choose to spend her last days in a hospice. She doesn't want aggressive treatment if there is clearly no way back. She would like to be kept comfortable and out of pain, even in the case that increasing pain relief will have the effect of shortening her life. It gives her some peace of mind to know that her husband and children won't need to argue or try to guess what she would want. Linda likes the idea of being a wise old woman, of passing on what she knows to her children and grandchildren – something she tries to do in her conversations with them, and in the letters she's written for them to read after she's gone. I felt I was benefiting from the warmth of Linda's wisdom too, reassured by the possibility that as you near death, the mind can tend towards a reconciliation with your own end.

Part of the trick seemed to be to look at death the right amount, neither too little nor too much. Linda had long ago stopped pushing her thoughts of death down and away. She had looked death square in the face; it seemed doing so had freed her to return her attention to life in the present moment.

Both John and Linda both told me that focusing on what they still have, despite the limitations of illness, imbued their lives with continuing joy and meaning. MSA has made John's world smaller and slower, but this mode of living comes with pleasures of its own. John told me walking his dog in the woods remained one of his delights on a daily basis, the new-found leisure of retirement allowed him to enjoy discussion groups through his local U3A and he was taking satisfaction from his key role in the lives of his grandchildren. Linda was relishing her tight-knit book group, her re-adoption of portrait painting and her interactions – online and in person – with others holding values similar to her own. In conversation with Robert McCrum for his memoir on mortality, *Every Third Thought*, psychotherapist Adam Philips suggested that ageing should not be thought of as the loss of youth: 'Ageing is ageing. Every stage of the life cycle is potentially interesting. And it's particularly interesting if you don't think of it elegiacally, if you don't think "what have I lost?" but instead, "what can I do now?"' John and Linda were both consciously placing this second question at the driving heart of their lives. This is part of the answer about how to live well given the fact of death: stop fixating on the story's ending and just enjoy the part of the story you are living in now. It's obvious, of course, but I seemed to need to hear this answer repeatedly to begin to feel convinced.

Linda told me that to dwell too much on fears of death poisons the experience of daily living. In the end we're all going to go – 'It doesn't matter how anxious people are, how frightened, it will happen in the end.' I came to understand that Linda had looked at death in a way that was useful to her – recognising its inevitability, she has made practical preparations. But the way I have looked at death – too much, without acceptance and with no constructive practical outcome – had not been useful to me. That thought has stuck with me – I shouldn't uselessly waste my life in rumination. The non-religious believe in no hereafter; this life here and now is what we have. I know I'm lucky there is so much in my here and now that's good.

During Linda's telling of her story to me, there was only one point at which she lost composure for a moment. It was when she imagined her children in a world without her in it. Linda's wish is Dale and Sally will be rooted in their own networks strongly enough that nothing will collapse when she goes. She is very close to them, they both seek her advice still. She choked a little telling me she sometimes wonders if she should pull away a bit, to help ready them for life without her. Our babies are still our babies even when they're in their fifties. We want them to be ok; and we'll always want to know what happens next for them. Death can never fully be a tying up of loose ends; it cuts the story off mid-sentence. Her children, her grandchildren are the main reasons Linda wants to continue living - but they are also the reasons she feels ok to go.

What came through most strongly, in what both John and Linda had to say, was the fulfilment they found, living in the warm centre of a loving family group. Their daily lives were made up of frequent, mutually-enjoyable interactions with those they loved most. Each was in a solidly supportive partnership of several decades standing. They'd raised children, and continued to have a hand in raising grandchildren who would take parts of them forward into the future – their genes, their memories, their values. I hope to feel this kind of intimate connectedness when I reach my own final chapters. But I wondered too, about those living a different kind of life. For those more socially isolated, what can mitigate the cold, hard fact of death? Meeting Matthew helped me begin to answer that.

8

MATTHEW

looking inward and reaching outward

When Matthew first got his prostate cancer diagnosis at the age of 69, he'd just spent two weeks with his dearest cousin as she died of cancer. He lives in London, but his cousin Gail was living in South Africa, where Matthew had himself grown up. Gail's daughter called and said 'Look, Mum's dying and we want you to be here, can you come?' Gail was surrounded by her children and grandchildren and they were giving her so much love. She wasn't fighting what was coming. She'd been told she only had six weeks, and by the time Matthew arrived, some of those weeks had already gone by. So she knew it, the children knew it, no one had to hide the fact that she was dying and it was good to have that in the open. Gail was peaceful about it, there was no angst, and she was so happy that Matthew had flown over to be there. She was totally compos mentis up until her last two days. Then, on the morphine drip, she slipped into a coma and faded, faded to the end. Matthew thought, *dying's not so difficult. I won't be surrounded by the children I don't have, perhaps I won't even want my friends around, I don't know. But it doesn't look so hard.* Matthew doesn't fear death. He's seen many friends dying, first from AIDS and more recently it's been mainly cancer.

When Matthew's biopsy confirmed a diagnosis of advanced localised prostate cancer, the consultant told him, 'Well, you've got to have a prostatectomy, you've got to have radiotherapy.' But Matthew thought *what have I really got to live for? I haven't got a family, I haven't had a partner for many years, I'm alone.* He thought he'd let the cancer take him. He said no to surgery, no to radiation. He did agree to hormone therapy – a testosterone blocker that slows the cancer's growth. He thought perhaps he'd have two years, to do a bit more travelling, and that would be fine.

Matthew was born to a Catholic father and Protestant mother who split when he and his younger brother were still very small. In theory, the boys were in their mother's custody, but she moved across the country for a job, and in any case was always on her own search for love. The two of them were dispatched to a convent boarding school. It made Matthew feel special to be chosen as an altar boy; he'd to ring the bells at certain points, swing the incense, and say the responses in Latin during Mass. The chapel had a marble altar draped in gorgeous satins and gold-threaded stuff. In the quadrangle the nuns had an incredible flower garden, and vases of cut roses would be all around. There were statues, candelabra, stained glass windows. Matthew loved the singing and the mystery of the Latin chanting. There was beauty, for his eyes and ears and nose. (The woman who lives in the flat below Matthew now, burns that same incense and it takes him back. He'd like to burn some himself but has been warned it would set his smoke alarm off, which makes a racket, so he doesn't.) Of course, on top of the sensory feast, was the religion. Jesus loves you and there are saints up there - Matthew got really into all that. They gave the kids comic books, in which the superheroes were the forty martyrs who sacrificed their lives and went straight up to God. Matthew wanted to be a martyr, too. He soaked up the magic and the romance, because what else did he have? For a child who didn't get parental love, God and Mary were there to fill that gap. The convent school was mainly for girls and there were no boys older than about eleven. On the evening of his last day, Matthew went into the chapel alone. The candlelight was glowing red through the glass of the tabernacle lamp, a sign of God's presence. Matthew was sad he wouldn't be coming back to this place. He knelt and said to God, 'If you will make my father well, I will become a priest.'

Matthew's father was a drunkard, who according to his mother kept defaulting on the alimony, and whom he saw probably three times in his entire childhood. On one occasion, Matthew and his brother visited their father. He didn't have his own place and the three of them had to share a bed. Matthew woke to his father having an epileptic fit, and no other adults in the house to call on. 'God' didn't make him better. Not that day, but some years down the line, 'God' took Matthew's father, so neither of his father figures turned out of much use to him. By the time his father died, though, Matthew had already parted ways, first with Catholicism and then with God. In the convent school, before bedtime, the nuns would get the children to line up for bathing. You'd take off shoes and socks, then wrap your towel round you while you took your trousers off. Then you got handed a kind of plastic skirt and went through to the bathroom where a nun would wash you with the skirt still on. So what was underneath that plastic skirt? You'd no idea. You were not connected to your body. Of course, as he got older, Matthew couldn't help but become aware of what was going on down there. He'd been told a guardian angel was on one shoulder and the devil on the other. He began having thoughts of the kind you shouldn't have if you don't want to burn in hell. But how do you stop them? In any case, Matthew liked those thoughts, and he liked it when, at around 12, at his second boarding school, he and another boy went for a long walk holding hands and touched each other through their clothes. If he wanted to take communion, he'd have to go to confession, but he thought *no, I don't see why,* so he stopped going to the Catholic church.

For a while, he looked for God elsewhere. He had the right to a British passport because his father's family had come from Scotland. So, at 16, he worked his way to London on a Merchant Navy ship, and stayed with a friend of a friend until he found his feet. He made Jewish friends and went to synagogue with them; he tried Buddhism and Rosacrucianism and it was *oh, I like this bit, don't like that bit,* for a while. Matthew began work as assistant resident warden, in a home for young people who were in those days called mentally handicapped or subnormal. One morning, he woke up with the distinct thought *God is dead.* It was the usual thing – *why so much suffering?* These were young men between around 15 and 22, who had been plonked in institutions from an early age because their parents couldn't cope. They were of an age the world should have been opening up for them – as it was for Matthew at the time – but their world didn't go beyond the walls of this place. Matthew'd been questioning, *who would – why would you want to do this* and reached the conclusion that this world isn't guided by a supreme, moral being. No more God for him.

For a long time, Matthew was timid about his atheism; it became another aspect of himself he didn't mention. He'd grown up with a secret in his head – homosexuality was diabolical according to Catholicism, and still illegal in South Africa. Matthew never told anyone in his family he was gay. The word 'moffie,' meaning queer, was freely traded as an insult in his uncles' homes. Then when he came to London with his South African accent, at a time when apartheid was facing increasing criticism, Matthew quickly learnt it was better to say he was from Wales, and later managed to develop quite a convincing Cockney accent. As a child, Matthew had not been housetrained in a social way, and he became an adult who habitually held others at a distance. He found it difficult to form close relationships, and many of the friends he did make have died over the years.

After his cancer diagnosis, Matthew struggled with the shock of seeing himself as a person with a serious illness. Until then, he'd always been a fit and healthy man. Now he felt vulnerable and all the more alone, because this wasn't stuff he could talk about with friends. He has a few close friends, including Ted and Reggie, but they're older than him and dealing with health problems of their own. When he visits, he puts on his bright and happy face and that makes them bright and happy too. A local cancer care centre offered a counselling service. Matthew saw the counsellor and vroom! It all came out. That was a relief and helped him to connect some dots with what he was feeling.

In the early days of diagnosis, Matthew would sometimes get on a train to the Southwest coast, with just his camera. He'd go for long walks on the cliffs, alone with the butterflies and birds. He remembers sitting looking down at the vast expanse of water thinking *isn't life strange and wonderful. What does it feel like to be part of the ocean, part of the sky? Because we are, aren't we? And we will be when we die.* He found that soothing. He found himself drawn to deserted places. Whenever he went somewhere new, he'd seek out derelict buildings and feel at home in them somehow. He'd photograph the emptiness, broken down walls, and the reflections on the standing water. Matthew had always been a keen photographer; he digitised the stacks of photos he'd amassed over the decades, when it seemed that film would become obsolete. Now he began to look back through pictures from the eighties. Matthew was in his forties then and still felt young. He was living in Durban and had bought an expensive underwater camera to use while scuba diving in the ocean. He thought he'd capture lovely images of fishes and coral. But shots had to be focused and f-stops calculated, which it turned out was not so easy when you're being swept along by currents and trying to avoid sharks.

At the time, Matthew was running an agency, training men to dance at hen parties. (It was amazing – the guys would do their stuff and you'd think they were Hollywood stars, the ladies loved it!) Some of the guys thought they'd also like to do some modelling and Matthew photographed them for their portfolios. Then he had the idea of using his underwater camera in the seawater pool at the beachfront, so a few guys came along for that. When he looks back at those pictures now – at the sunlight playing on young bodies, gliding under water as if in flight – it reminds him life can be good, as it was then. *God, when I was doing this I'd no idea!* He'd felt invincible, like nothing could tear his world apart. Life was happy and creative, fuelled by the enthusiasm and love of many wonderful friends. Then one friend,

Bruce, got an ulcer on his leg that wouldn't heal. For a long time, Bruce didn't tell Matthew what was wrong; there was a series of episodes when Bruce would get sick and hide himself away, and Matthew would find his friend and help put him back together. Then he stopped hearing from Bruce; Bruce didn't answer his phone or his door and someone living in the same block told Matthew Bruce was in the hospital. When Matthew went in to see him, Bruce was far gone with AIDS, unable to speak, and died about 10 days later. Matthew said to himself after that, *I've always been promiscuous – if I were to contract HIV, I would be spreading it.* He decided *that's it: celibate.* That was 30 years ago.

Sex was still in the brain, though, till he started the testosterone blocker to slow his cancer. Matthew attended a conference for men with prostate cancer, about how to stay as healthy as possible while on hormone treatment. He was asked to write a report about the day for a newsletter. A while later, reflecting on thoughts of then and now, he had the idea to superimpose some of the words about the prostate cancer conference onto his underwater swimming images. Fragments of text float over weightless forms: '… physiotherapy team managed to get us off our chairs,' '… and live longer,' '… an erection which can be maintained, with a rubber seal at the base of the cock, when the pump is removed.' Bringing pictures from then and words from now together is Matthew's way of saying his cancer can't blot out the joy and the vitality that have been his.

Coming up to two years after diagnosis, entering a new year, Matthew realised *I still feel quite well, ok, I have cancer, but why not make the best of it? If this year could be my last, let's make it the best year ever!* He planned trips to Paris and Madrid, up and down the UK. He was awarded a few thousand pounds following a lawsuit about his leaky roof. That gave him a bit of leeway to plan trips, without needing to worry too much about the cost. Matthew loves the whole project of a trip. As soon as he decides to go somewhere, he'll be totally involved – choosing where to stay and working out how he'll get there. He'll have an envelope marked, say, 'Manchester,' and he'll start to fill it up with info, maps and information about exhibitions that are coming on. Whenever he goes away, he feels a different person. It's as if there's no cancer, no hang-ups, he can just be an explorer and it's wonderful. Then when he's back there's the project of putting the best shots in a photobook. He buys discounted credits online, and at one point paid for 30 in advance that had to be completed within three months, so that kept him busy for a while! Matthew likes the way a project with a fixed timeframe gives him a structure to work within. He would hate to live forever. *How boring and how lonely*, he thinks. The cancer diagnosis gave an urgency to Matthew's time – it was its own kind of project with a deadline, and there was excitement in that.

The photobook he's proudest of is probably the one of Birmingham. Matthew used sometimes to look at friends who've had successful lives and regret he hasn't had a real career to look back on. He hoped he'd get to the point with his photographs of saying 'This is what I've done, guys.' He thought he could die happy if a gallery picked up his work and said, 'We'll do a show,' or a publisher said 'Hey look, we'll do a book.' He had six of his best shots from the Birmingham photobook printed; the idea was to send them to Birmingham City Council and say 'Hey, what do you think of this?' If at least they wrote him back a little letter, he could try to sell his book on Amazon with a note saying Birmingham City Council say 'These pictures are interesting.' But Matthew hasn't sent the pictures. And now? There is no longer time for looking back, regretting. The past is simply everything that's brought him to the point where he is now; he tries to focus on the present and the future that remains.

Around that two-year post-diagnosis mark, Matthew was having pains in his leg and went for osteopathic treatment. The osteopath was a young Italian guy, Antonio. Taking testosterone-blockers can thin the bones and weaken muscles, so Antonio suggested Matthew would benefit from swimming and going to the gym. Matthew said he'd think about it. At the next session, Antonio had made a list of swimming pools, how much they cost, how far they were away. Matthew thought *this is amazing – why would someone do that for me?* And so he chose a pool, went up there, joined. By that point in his treatment, he had developed boobs, so he decided to go swimming with a t-shirt on.
    The lifeguard said 'You can't come in with that on.'
    'Why?'
    'It's the regulation.'
    'I don't believe this!'
    'Well, not unless you've got a medical condition.'
Matthew explained about his cancer and they let him through. The next time it was a different lifeguard so he had to go through it all again, and so on. Until Antonio presented him with one of those latex swim tops that professional divers wear. Matthew thought then, *this is kindness, beyond.* Apart from that, Matthew thought, as Antonio went through a series of gentle manipulations, *I can feel something coming from his hands.* When he goes to visit Ted and Reggie on a Saturday, there are the religious people out on the high street with their Bibles. As people pass by they ask 'Do you need healing?' Sometimes, they'll have someone's head in their hands, and they'll be asking Jesus to heal that person. For Matthew, there's no Jesus, but he believes there *is* something that happens between people when they touch

each other. At one point in the eighties, when his friends were dying from AIDS and Matthew began to think more about what it means to be well, he trained as a masseur. There was all this research around – why were kids in orphanages dying, though they were being fed and kept in a clean environment? And what was special about one particular institution where the children thrived? It was that they were touched. They were picked up and cuddled.

Matthew thought *I'm lucky to have survived my childhood because I don't remember being held or stroked by anyone.* With Antonio, Matthew felt, *this is an empathetic human being, these are the actions, these are the hands of someone who cares.* At Christmas time, Matthew gave Antonio a copy of his Birmingham photobook as a present. A few weeks later, Antonio said 'By the way, my mother called – she's been looking through your photobook, she loves it! She checked out your website, too.' To Matthew, this was overwhelming – that an Italian mama somewhere had taken the trouble and seen something in the images he'd made. Knowing Antonio cared what happened to him made Matthew care more about himself. It was a turning point. He began to work determinedly in the pool and at the gym to maintain strength and flexibility.

When Antonio mentioned his mother had looked at Matthew's website, it was wonderful to hear, but also made Matthew disappointed with himself, because he hadn't put up any new pictures on the site for a long time and had done nothing with the photos from his latest Paris trip. He noticed his enthusiasm to make something of his photography had drained away. For a while he kept taking photos out of habit; then suddenly thought *why are you bothering when you aren't doing anything with them?* He has to sort of stroke himself and say 'Well, you're not superman, you're just a lonesome guy.' When he thought about it more, he realised his photography had been a solitary occupation. If he takes over a photobook, Ted and Reggie are complimentary, but it's not their thing. In the last ten years, five of Matthew's closest friends have died – Richard, Adrian, Gail, Chris, Estella. They're not around him any more, to listen or tell him about their own projects; he's lost that energising interchange. The solitary walks, the focus on making images that held meaning – these activities helped him come to terms with loss. People who'd been important to him were gone, and with his illness, he was losing aspects of himself, too.

But now Matthew began to notice something shifting in himself. He noticed when he went to Paris, how people acknowledge each other. Even getting into a lift, you say 'Bonjour, Madame,' and you'll always get a response. That happens less in London. Now, on the tube, if someone smiles, Matthew will smile back. Even better if he's the one that smiles first and gets an answering smile. The first prostate cancer support group Matthew joined didn't work for him. It was run by a woman and some of the men came with their wives. There was a reluctance to call a spade a spade: people shied away from plain talk about what was happening to their penises. When he joined the group specifically for gay men with prostate cancer, Matthew felt relieved to be able to speak more freely.

Then, he joined a choir for people with cancer, at his local Maggie's cancer centre. You start off as a room full of strangers. The session begins with warm-up exercises that involve making faces at each other, so already you relax and smile. And then, you know you've all got cancer, so that's something in common. There are more women than men at the choir. The way the women at choir have talked easily to Matthew about their feelings has helped him to open up as well. He's bonding with the men there, too. You sit next to a guy, and it's 'Well, what hospital are you at?' 'How far along with your treatment are you?' 'How are you today?' Before the practice sessions, you could have tea and biscuits. Matthew noticed people were coming earlier and earlier each week to chat; a community was forming. It's a lovely place. As soon as you go in, a volunteer will welcome you and say 'What can I get you?' In the winter, there's a lovely big fire, where you can pull up a chair and feel at home.

It's been five years now since Matthew's diagnosis. The testosterone-blockers he was taking stopped working, and he had to move on to injections that stop his body from producing testosterone entirely, so he has hot flushes and night sweats to deal with now. Sooner or later the cancer will find a way of feeding itself again, and then a new regime will need to be considered. But he'd have to say he's had five good years, and, looking around at choir practice, he sees many others haven't been as lucky. That makes him grateful to be still relatively able and mobile. It feels good, too, that he can be there for others who are having a tough time. If he sees someone looking sad, he'll give that person a hug; he'll take them aside and ask how they are doing. Being in the choir has loosened Matthew up. He cares more about other people now, and less about how others may judge him. With groups he's been part of in the past, he's turned down invitations to the pub, for fear of questions: 'Wife? Kids?' They may have been ok with Matthew's answers to these, but he preferred not risk it. At the choir group, they take each other as they are, and Matthew feels comfortable to be himself. It seems the group gets tighter each week – when people go on holiday they'll put up photos on WhatsApp and they'll stay in touch if someone can't come to practice because of chemo. The concerts bind the choir members closely – you get nervous and excited with each other.

One of the concerts, held in a local church, was a celebration of the music of famous singers who had died: George Michael, David Bowie, and finishing with Leonard Cohen's 'Hallelujah.' The audience were exhorted to join in with the chorus. Hallelujah, hallelujah... the word can be translated 'praise the Lord.' Doubtless, many of those singing in the church that evening, facing the travails of cancer, shared Matthew's disbelief in any God whom we should praise. And yet, as the choir members stood shoulder to shoulder with each other, face to face with those who'd come to listen and support, it was clear in the notes rising amongst them all that something special was happening.

9

ON JOINING SONG

secular community and connection

Early in the forming of this book, my online searches repeatedly returned headlines declaring religious people happier than non-religious people. I wondered whether that was really true. I noticed most of the studies behind the headlines were coming out of the USA, a Christian-majority country. It makes sense that in a country where non-religiosity still carries some stigma, those who can comfortably belong within prevailing social norms may on average be happier than those who can't. I discovered, however, that in places where religious believers are in the minority, such as the Netherlands and Denmark, there's no significant correlation between religiosity and happiness. Roy Speckhardt, executive director of the American Humanist Association, has also pointed out that many US studies have equated being 'highly religious' with frequent attendance of religious services, an approach which 'doesn't measure the differences between the religious and the nonreligious, but instead measures the difference between those that have strong community connections and those that do not.' He argued that it is not religion, but community that has positive outcomes.

A subsequent study of 26 countries (not including the UK) lends support to this view: the 'inactively religious' (those claiming a religious identity but only infrequently attending services) weren't happier than the 'religiously unaffiliated' (those who don't identify with any organised religion.) But the 'actively religious' (those regularly attending services) were the happiest group studied. The regular interactions of the 'actively religious' with likeminded others may build a secure sense of belonging and offer a supportive network to lean on during tough times. But in the UK today, only 18% of people attend religious services at least monthly. The great majority of us aren't 'actively religious' and more than half of us are non-religious. So what does that mean for our happiness?

As we get older or become unwell, social networks we've previously relied on can become strained and ruptured. We may be stepping away from the world of work; gaping holes may appear in the fabric of our lives as more of our friends and relatives die. We may find ourselves isolated and lonely just at those times when we could do with more support. Having social support is associated with better psychological well-being amongst patients suffering from a wide range of chronic illnesses, such as cancer, coronary heart disease and diabetes. Conversely, loneliness is associated with increased depression, heightened blood pressure and a weakened immune system; loneliness is as detrimental to health as smoking or substance abuse.

I became interested in the possibility that belonging to a Godless congregation could boost the happiness of non-religious people and might help us weather the storms of loss, ageing and illness. One morning in 2018, Andy Pakula told me how he came be the non-religious minister of a north London congregation, and about the community he's helped build.

At some mid-life point, the thought began to emerge more insistently for Andy, *I don't want my tombstone to say "Here lies Andy: he went to a lot of meetings and made some rich investors richer."* Raised in suburban New York, he'd so far swallowed what the dominant culture told him – that you're supposed to get a good job and make a lot of money, so you can buy a big suburban home and give your 1.5 kids all the stuff they want. Andy studied at MIT, got into biotech, was climbing up that ladder. Then when he and his wife had a son, they wanted him to grow up within some kind of community. Someone said 'Oh, the Unitarians take atheists,' so they went along; they liked what they experienced at the Unitarian Universalist church, which was less about God and more about people being together.

It was in his mid-40s that Andy became increasingly cynical about biotech and more interested in what was going on in the congregation at church. Most of the time, people will put on a brave face and give the world a smile, automatically answer 'fine' when someone asks them how they're doing. Growing up and as a younger man, Andy had never really had the opportunity to be in deep community, where people are honest about what's going on. He'd believed people's inner lives are like the surface that they show. He'd had the sense *everyone is happy, except me.* Now, as a member of the Unitarian Universalist congregation, it was a huge relief to him to realise we're not alone with this, we all feel shitty sometimes. It wasn't an easy thing for Andy to jump down from the high career rung he'd climbed to and find himself at the bottom of a different ladder. He did it, though, and wound up here: as an atheist church minister in north London. Unitarianism is in decline, but Andy's congregation, New Unity, has grown five-fold since he took over here in 2010 and is now the largest Unitarian congregation in Britain. So, New Unity is offering something people want. At the services, there's communal singing, live music, readings, reflection on an ethical topic, candle-lighting. It's not for everyone – to some atheists and humanists, the thought of any kind of church experience is queasy-making. Others, though, who have no use for God do still want the chance to connect deeply.

One of the means through which connection happens at New Unity is the ritual of candles of joy and sorrow. Each week, members of the congregation are invited up to light a candle for a joy or sorrow they are carrying. They may do this silently, but most will share something aloud. It could be, 'I'm pregnant,' or 'My dad's been diagnosed with dementia.' It's life, it's all the life things, and it helps create an environment where people feel safe to share what's really going on for them. One week Kirsty, a woman in her early thirties, lit a candle and said 'I had a brain tumour but it's out and I'm really glad about that.' Afterwards, people went up to her and hugged her. She knew no matter what the community would support her – emotionally, and, if needed, practically too. She belonged. Initially, Kirsty's breast cancer had appeared to be treatable. When later it was found to have spread significantly, Andy agreed with Kirsty that it sucked she was going to die. Then he asked 'What do you want to do with the time you have remaining?' She said 'I want to get married and I want to work with a cancer charity.' And she did it – she got on the board of a charity that was doing great stuff and used her skills from marketing to help them take things further. She was single at the time of diagnosis, but she met someone, they fell in love and married. They ran off to Scotland to do it quickly, but later they were able to have a wedding blessing, with Andy officiating.

She knew she had a handful of years at best, and she really focused on what brought joy and meaning to her life. People would tell her 'You're so courageous' and she'd reply, 'I'm not – this is just the life I have.' She inspired people, though; others were uplifted by their connection to her, as she was by hers to them. A couple in the community named their child after her, and it was a joyful moment when Kirsty held that child in her arms.

Andy visited her in hospice, where she spent the last weeks of her life. The two of them had an honest conversation. Kirsty really had reconciled herself to dying; for her, the physical discomfort was the worst part of what she was experiencing. Friends often find it hard not to try to fix stuff, but not everything can be fixed. A pastoral carer can sit with a person and hold the pain. There was space for lightness, too. Kirsty lit a cigarette: 'I'm dying - I can smoke if I want!'

A lot of the support within the New Unity community happens informally. Friendships form organically, people exchange texts and go for coffees. Sometimes, people may benefit from support that's offered in a more formal and structured way. There's a pastoral care team; initially, Andy trained the pastoral carers, in line with the core principles of the humanist psychologist Carl Rogers. It's about unconditional positive regard. Whatever someone says, you aren't going to think less of them, you aren't going to judge or run away. If someone is struggling, a member of the pastoral care team can contact them in private and say 'Would you like to talk?' Typically, a member of the team will meet someone up to six times; it's a chance for that person to unburden themselves and have someone really listen. There are also groups that have been set up for mutual support – including a men's group and a women's group. It's very intergenerational, with members from their twenties to their eighties. People can share what's going on for them, share thoughts, share food.

Andy thinks it's valuable for younger people to get a sense what life is like as you get older. He has in common with other church ministers that he sees his community as standing against the evils of the world. For him, though, unlike for many religious ministers, gay marriage is a good; and it would be progress, in Andy's view, to allow people more power to choose the manner of their own death. One of the evils against which Andy tries to stand, though, is the ageism inherent in modern Western culture. So, he was delighted when a congregation member approached him about helping her celebrate an important milestone: her 60th birthday. She wanted to bring together friends and relations to mark her transition to a new phase. If Julia had recently been born, was reaching adulthood, getting married, or had just died, Andy would have known what to do. The transition from adult to elder, though, is rarely celebrated. Together, she and Andy planned a fitting ceremony. When the evening came, Andy welcomed those gathered for Julia, and told them they were there not to console, but to rejoice with Julia in the new opportunities that lay ahead. They sang together, gave Julia gifts and words of love. Jenny Joseph's 'Warning' was read aloud – a poem outlining plans for an irresponsible old age, to include wearing purple with a garish red hat and growing fat on sausages. Maturity confers us the freedom to shed the inhibitions of our self-conscious youth. We can grow stronger, more confident in our own skin, even as that skin thins and wrinkles. Andy led those present in a ritual to honour Julia's symbolic journey into elderhood. He asked for those under the age of 60 to stand at one end of the room, those over 60 at the other. Julia stood first with the youngers, who promised to remain her loved ones through all of her changes. The elders promised to hold Julia and share with her what they'd learned. And then, Julia crossed the room to join them. Andy brought the ceremony to a close with words about the way our lives trace a path through the world, and how at each stage – childhood, youth, adulthood and the elder years – we can embrace our opportunities to grow and shine.

Looking at the New Unity community under Andy's leadership, I saw how a group of people can be bonded not by faith in God, but by other elements traditionally associated with religious communities: by song, ritual, and a commitment to shared moral values. This was a strong, warm community that had supported its member Kirsty through the joys and sorrows of life with terminal cancer; it was also a community that overtly celebrated members of all ages and stages of life. I admired the non-religious community Andy was helping to establish.

And he wasn't the only one. In January 2013, a few years after Andy Pakula took on leadership of New Unity's non-religious congregations, comedians Pippa Evans and Sanderson Jones launched the first Sunday Assembly in London, having discovered they shared a desire to be part of a church-like form of community, but without any supernatural element. Under the motto 'live better, help often, wonder more,' The Sunday Assembly experience involves listening to speakers and readings intended to inspire congregants to live their own lives fully and support each other. Communal singing, often of upbeat pop music, is also a key feature of Sunday Assembly gatherings. The Sunday Assembly concept has caught on; there are now satellite congregations in more than 40 locations worldwide, of which 18 are in the UK. Sunday Assembly has raised awareness that people can come together to sing, think and support each other, without a belief in God being the ticket to get in. Though the Sunday Assembly atmosphere is upbeat, there's an underlying awareness that life can be tough. During one assembly held in London, with the theme of Grief, Sanderson Jones said it was losing his mum at the age of 10 that led him to understand how precious and short life is, and ultimately inspired him to bring people together to celebrate life. It is part of the organisation's stated mission that every Sunday Assembly should be a place of compassion, where those who are socially isolated are welcomed, and those with worries can find solace.

This is all lovely, but… When Andy Pakula acknowledged that the church-like experience of New Unity and Sunday Assembly is not for everyone, and that for some atheists and humanists the idea of being in 'deep community' is 'queasy-making,' I understood what he meant, because, honestly, it's a bit queasy-making for me. I've been to New Unity and Sunday Assembly services, and to local humanist meetings. On these occasions, part of me was recognising *these are nice, good people and there are nice, good things happening,* but another part of me was thinking *get me out of here!* It is partly that, as an introvert, I find group interactions in general difficult. Also, Richard Dawkins' oft-quoted statement springs to mind: organising atheists is 'like herding cats.' Those who reject organised religion are often rejecting both the organised and the religion elements equally.

Having been pushed into giving up work by the encroaching symptoms of multiple systems atrophy, John, whom we met in chapter 4, was enjoying some aspects of his retirement, including the lively discussions of the U3A groups he'd joined. He liked that he shared similar interests with the other members, but also that they didn't always agree on everything. John speculated that, though raised by two devout parents, somehow a gene (or several) had slipped through that told him to question everything all the time. Having given his local humanist group a try, he decided not to continue going. For him, the humanist meetings had 'the same atmosphere that my parents' Baptist chapel did when I was a kid, all this enthusiastic devoutness.' There was a sense of 'We all think the same way, don't we?' and 'We're all humanists because…' John felt an inner resistance to this group think.

In some ways a similar character to John, Simon told me that something inside puts him at least 50% on the defensive at any social gathering. In his boarding school days, Simon used to attend chapel every Sunday. At 89 when I met him, he had long ago dismissed all that God stuff as bogus, but he was still seeking to connect with others on Sundays. The trouble was, the friends he'd had at school – how could he put this in a way that wasn't too pompous? – well, he'd outgrown them. And the other thing was, they were all dead. He'd made new, younger friends, but they were often busy, they had other things to do. On Sundays though, Simon noted, some people do still gather, and sometimes he liked to be among them. In the previous three months he'd tried the Methodists, the Unitarians, and Quakers, as well as his local C of E church. He'd usually tell these people 'I'm an agnostic I'm afraid,' and they'd be very nice and say it doesn't matter and that they hoped he'd come back next week. Usually, he did go back a second time, because that welcome, that goodwill drew him in. Usually, he didn't go back a third or fourth time, because he hadn't found his tribe.

Simon and I stayed in touch after I interviewed him. I suggested we go together to a Sunday Assembly service. I was interested to see what he would make of it.

At the service, the two of us sit together near the front, as Simon is hard of hearing. When asked who's attending for the first time, I raise my hand and get a high five, but Simon doesn't raise his – he says later he only caught about 30% of what was said. He's been in a room with a couple of hundred happy people, and there's something nice in that, but he found it an uncomfortable experience. He feels situationally freakish as one of the last ones standing of his generation. Watching girls in very short shorts dancing on the stage, he was wondering *what will they think if they look my way?* '*What's that old guy doing here? He can't rave like I can.*' After the service, Simon tells me he didn't feel able to share in the good feelings of the gathering – the poppy music didn't register with him, he wasn't able to connect. As he tells me this, we're sitting on a bench outside the building where, inside, attendees are still engaged in clustered chatter. I ask if Simon would like to go back in, but he doesn't want to, he doesn't think he could get anywhere with the people inside. For my part, I'm glad of the excuse Simon has supplied me to walk away myself – away from those who've gathered to commune and to connect. I suppose John, Simon and I are each that kind of cat that resists being herded. I am the cat that likes to crouch, concealed, alert, watching and listening. Like John, there's something in me that bristles at the threat of being absorbed into a 'like-minded' group.

*

When I first met Matthew, he told me he was a very independent person. He doesn't find it easy to be with others – even friends – for any length of time and is reluctant to accept offers of help. He hadn't been 'housetrained' as a child in a social way. He was raised without parental care and guidance, dispatched to boarding school, and then the need to hide his sexuality made it habitual in him to keep others at a distance. Loneliness can become a habit that is tough to break. As we go further into ourselves, it becomes harder to reach out to others. But a year and a bit later, Matthew told me he'd registered an inner shift: 'I used to call myself an antisocial person…' He was, by that point, a member of not one, but five choirs. He was getting together to sing with others four days every week – on one day he'd go straight from one choir on a bus to the next. His life was full of music.

During our first conversation, Matthew told me how his diagnosis with prostate cancer coincided with the death of his cousin, Gail, to whom he had been close. He needed to take some time to look inwards; through walking alone in nature and in urban settings, photographing what he saw, and organising those images in photobooks, Matthew was gradually able to make some sense of his situation and his feelings. Then, the experience of feeling supported by an empathetic osteopath was a turning point for Matthew. He tentatively began to reach out to others who could support him, and to whom he could offer support. When the first prostate cancer support group that he attended wasn't quite a fit, Matthew found another group, specifically for gay men, which offered him more. One day, with another guy, he went along to a prostate cancer road show. They heard from various medical professionals about developments in the prostate cancer world, and someone from the Royal College of Music came round saying they were going to form a choir, in collaboration with the Welsh charity Tenovus, because research shows singing together is particularly beneficial for cancer patients and their families. Singing together can forge rapid bonds between erstwhile strangers and can help alleviate anxiety and depression. Since Tenovus launched its first 'Sing With Us' choir in 2010, choir members have been uplifted by song, and by belonging to a community of people who have been through, or are going through similar experiences. Matthew and his friend both signed up for the new London 'Sing with Us' choir.

At the start of the first session he went to, the choir leader had everyone doing warm-up exercises, pulling funny faces, had Matthew sticking out his tongue at perfect strangers. You can't help smiling and relaxing. And that helps you start to talk and open up. Matthew was thinking *this is more of a support group than all of the support groups I've been to before.* And he'd always loved to sing, since his days as a boy chorister. Tenovus, at the time, were funding further research on the benefits of singing in a choir for mental health and wellbeing. The researchers were out recruiting more participants for the study, so new people kept showing up to rehearsals. 50 or more people were coming to choir each week. For Matthew it was getting to feel too big and too much flux. Then someone told him they were also a member of another, very small and lovely choir at the local Maggie's cancer centre. He went along to Maggie's, liked it a lot and stopped going to Tenovus after a while. Then a choir started at his gym and he went along. That's a group of people who are enthusiastic about keeping themselves healthy – the energy lifts Matthew up. Matthew decided to join a choral society too, and challenge his brain with learning songs in German, French and Latin. He joined a fourth choir focused mainly on basic training for the voice, and a fifth that does quite funky, jazzy stuff. It impressed me that Matthew, who had previously described himself as too shy and hung up to reach out to others, had gone all out in embracing group belonging. With an awareness of what did and didn't work for him, Matthew was recognising that sometimes it's worthwhile to push through initial discomfort towards the comfort of connection.

The members of Matthew's prostate cancer support group and of Maggie's choir were bound by the shared circumstance of illness. In *Staring at the Sun,* psychiatrist Irvin Yalom observes that the pain of knowing we must die can be tempered by our 'rich connections' to each other. He relays one woman's words during a group therapy session for people with terminal illnesses: 'It's a pitch black night. I'm alone in my boat floating in a harbour. I see the lights of many other boats. I know I can't reach them, can't join with them. But how comforting it is to see all those other lights bobbing in the harbour.' This image has stuck with me for the way it captures our alone-togetherness. There must remain an element of isolation in any person's experience of illness and dying; despite that, we can bob along together.

10

SOMEONE AT YOUR BEDSIDE

non-religious pastoral support, ii

Jane Flint was the first, and there still aren't many non-religious pastoral carers in paid roles within the NHS. In recent years, though, the Non-Religious Pastoral Support Network (NRPSN) has been training hundreds of volunteers, with the aim of providing access to non-religious pastoral support to anyone who needs it. Humanists UK were able to put me in touch with a number of hospital and hospice volunteers, who told me about the support they offer patients and their families in times of crisis.

Dennis visits his local hospital once a week. He sees how unnerving it is for people when they lose control of their lives. You're ill – which is why you're in hospital, and the hospital environment tends to strip people of agency. The nurses and doctors chop and change with the shifts, dash in and do things with you and don't actually sit down to explain what's going on. Patients often have a look of helplessness, but Dennis can be a friendly face. He may say, 'Still waiting to see the doctor, are you?' or 'How are you getting on?' If the patient answers 'Fine,' he'll say 'What are you doing here then?' which can often raise a smile. If he can leave people feeling a bit more relaxed and comfortable with their situation, because they've had a chance to talk about what's going on, Dennis feels he's being of some help.

When Eileen began volunteering, she was asked to shadow the hospital's C of E chaplain. She noticed he primarily targeted people who had attended the service at the hospital's chapel. There's never enough time to get round to everyone on the wards, so it seemed a little odd to Eileen that the chaplain was directing his support to those who'd already been able to go and find it for themselves. Now that Eileen can choose for herself whose beds to approach, she'll usually head first for people who are in a single room. If you're on a ward, there tends to be a lot going on, at least you've got stuff to look at, whereas being in a single room can be very isolating, especially if you're an infection risk and they've got to have the door closed. Eileen will put on the plastic gloves and apron and go to say hello. She often finds people sunk in misery, but they're nearly always delighted at the chance to chat, to have a bit of human contact. Eileen can listen, and by listening attentively, that then encourages the patient to expand – about their family, about positive experiences they've had – and the mood will lighten.

Heather volunteers at a hospice. One patient was hoping to make it to her granddaughter's wedding. Heather knew this lady was deteriorating and felt it was unlikely she'd live long enough to see the big day. She said, 'Let's hope you can get there, but just in case it isn't possible, would you like me to bring in some cards for you to choose from?' The patient said she'd like that, so Heather brought in a selection and the lady chose a card for her granddaughter, and another for her daughter. She couldn't be there on the day, as it turned out, but her granddaughter and daughter had the words from her she wanted them to have.

Howard also visits a hospice once a week. Most patients there have come in for end-of-life care. They're not surprised about it, and, when they have the energy for conversation, they often welcome a diversion, because dying can be a very tedious process. Howard may open by asking something like 'Is your wife coming to see you later?' Often that's a yes, and the conversation gets off on a positive note. Non-religious patients aren't thinking about whether they're going to a dark place or a bright one; they often want to look at what's already happened, rather than what's coming next. They appreciate the chance to tell you what they are and what they were. Howard has a lot of autobiographies lodged in his head. One guy had come from humble origins and gone on to become an international expert in skyscrapers. Often Howard only meets a patient once, but this guy he saw again the following week, and he could see the patient was pleased to see someone who already knew who he was, so that the conversation could carry on where they'd left off. Howard thinks there's real value in just being there, another human being to rub along with. That can be particularly important when someone doesn't have much in the way of support from family and friends. Howard is on the rota the hospice has set up, for patients who don't have anyone else to be with them at end-of-life. Those on the rota can each take a four-hour shift to be with that person. It might be holding their hand, or just making them aware you're there with them.

In 2018, Lindsay van Dijk became the first humanist to be appointed as lead chaplain by an NHS trust. When asked why it's essential hospitals offer non-religious pastoral support, she replied that patients often check with her, 'You're not religious, right?' because, 'for them, it's really important to have somebody like-minded to speak to before they feel comfortable enough to disclose the difficulties they're facing. Non-religious people, quite often, would rather speak to nobody than speak to a religious chaplain, so it's really important that they are heard.' When I first met Matthew, I asked him whether, if he were ill in hospital, he might be interested in speaking to a non-religious pastoral carer. He said he absolutely would. He has a good friend with strongly religious views, and usually he can deal with that ok, and enjoy the music, and the jumble sales he goes to at his friend's church. But, if he were very unwell and vulnerable, he wouldn't want to be approached by a religious chaplain. It would remind him of the damage done to him as a child, of being told he had the devil on his shoulder and was going to burn in hell.

If in the future I'm lying very unwell in a hospital or hospice bed, I can imagine I might welcome a conversation with someone like Jane, Lindsay, or a non-religious volunteer, too. I imagine also, that if the one lying in the bed isn't me but somebody I love, it would be a comfort to have someone at my side who sees things as I do, that death is really 'Goodbye' and not just 'See you soon.'

When I began this project, I was looking to speak to people facing their own mortality, due to old age or life-limiting illness. John, Linda, Matthew and many others each shared their perspective with me on how non-religious people can find happiness, hope and meaning up to the end of life. Some who offered to speak to me weren't facing the end of their own lives; they'd lost someone they dearly loved and wondered whether I might want to hear their stories. Of course I did. Louisa and many others told me about living through great loss.

11

LOUISA

the fact of happiness still stands

People ask Louisa whether she still talks to David, and she does – 'You bastard, where'd you hide that thing I need?' He'll always be the person that she *wants* to talk to. You lose your best friend, confidant and lover in one go. But she does not believe he hears her. Sometimes she'll go, 'On the off-chance you *can* hear me, this is what I'm thinking.' She hasn't gone so far as saying, 'Please give me a sign,' but if there were any way he could, she's sure he would. It's been eight months. And so he isn't, any longer, here.

Yet, in a thousand ways, he is. When they both knew he was very ill, he wrote down his passwords in a notebook. One day, she needs to get into a bank account, looks up the password and finds 'fuckmyoldboots,' so very David…She still comes across scraps of paper with his writing on, the backs of envelopes with his impromptu sketches and dimensions. On Facebook, things come up – '1 year ago' – with a picture of what they did that day, and she'll catch her breath. She shared a picture of their wedding on the anniversary and it had 74 likes. People she doesn't really know – friends of friends – are seeing it and reacting, and that feels sort of nice, a group hug somehow. Louisa likes looking at pictures of David. Though he was quite bloated from the steroids towards the end, that's not how she recalls him now. That most recent version of him was just a small percentage of their time, not their whole story, so it helps to look at earlier photographs as well. And she does have some nice shots from those last months too. The screensaver on David's computer is now of him on one of their last holidays, with the dog having just bounded out of view. David's face says something funny has just happened. Photos of the two of them together remind Louisa that nothing can take away the happiness – though short-lived – of the time they shared. The fact of their happiness still stands.

In a million ways, of course, he isn't here. It took her six months just to get rid of David's toothbrush, she couldn't take it out of the thing. And sometimes the photographs, the videos, feel like she's torturing herself. Because he had his kids and she had her daughter Jaz, they'd always kept both houses on; sometimes she catches herself thinking he's just at the other house… His birthday was hard, because she wasn't buying him a present, there was nothing to be done, and it felt very empty. His grown-up son told her that when Facebook reminded him to 'Wish David well!', he'd watched the video clip with his dad's voice twenty times or more. It's a couple of seconds of the dog wagging his tail and David's jaunty voice calling 'Harris, come on!' When there's something funny, Louisa resists the strong desire to text David. She has his phone here in the house; she would only be texting herself. It wouldn't help and so she doesn't do it. It's the intimacy of a secret language you miss. She's sent bits of humour to other people, but it's not the same, because they don't react how David would. It's not a gap that can be filled.

Some people have a list of places they'd like to go. Louisa and David had a list of places they really *didn't* want to go to. They'd be driving somewhere and hear a story on the radio about the dog-eating festivals in China or gay men being thrown off buildings in Saudi Arabia. And one of them would turn to the other and say, 'Shall we add it to the list?' They'd fantasise how they'd spend the money saved from not going to all those places. Louisa wanted wide oak floorboards and wildflower meadows. David wanted to restore a classic car and parp around the countryside like Toad of Toad Hall. There was a lot of sunshine, velvet and fine dining in these imaginings. Then, time, of course, came to seem so much more valuable than money. Think of all the time they saved not going to Dubai!… And now, when Louisa's driving and hears on the radio another story about North Korea, she wants to turn to David and say 'Already on the list,' but no one's there to turn to.

Louisa reached 50 not expecting to fall in love and all that stuff again, and yet it happened. The two of them agreed on almost everything, apart from the quantity of salt to put on food. She'd catch him adding extra salt to salted crisps. Louisa and David shared eight fantastic years; he died aged 66, four months after they got hitched. She called up the florist, saying, 'You know that wedding you did in September? Can you do the flowers for the funeral?' She'd asked David what he wanted for the funeral, no – she'd asked 'What *would* you want,' because it made it a bit easier to be theoretical. The closer you get to death, the harder it gets to look at it directly. He'd said, 'Absolutely no religion, beyond that, to be honest, I don't give a fuck, whatever you want.'

What Louisa wanted was a celebration of his life, and it was. She wore red. 100 people turned out, on a weekday, miles from anywhere. Of course, being January, the weather was foul; they drove up the motorway in pissing rain. Planning the day, Louisa had thought, *what are we going to do in a bloody field in January?* She would have to hire a marquee. She got a quote, which seemed a lot of money, so she phoned another place and haggled over price in a slightly embarrassed way, thinking, *well, I'm grieving but I'm not gullible!* She saved 800 quid for the sake of a phone call and thought, *you'd be proud of me, David!* Then on the day, it rained, so thank God for the marquee, where they had the readings, and the tribute.

It helped that the humanist celebrant guided Louisa through the structure of the day, telling her – 'It can be like this: you can have a reading, then a song, and then we'll go to the graveyard and say this.' He went to the trouble of really finding out about David from his ex-wives and business partners. It was as though David had lived enough for several lifetimes. The celebrant gathered all the stories from those different parts of David's life, to draw a picture of the whole man. One of David's friends said to Louisa later, 'We were at another funeral last week, someone we've known quite well for years. The vicar talked about this bloke we didn't even recognise.' Listening to the tribute to David, for Louisa was quite therapeutic. It was precious that these little snippets of David-before-she-knew-him should be recounted and preserved, shared with those who knew only their own bits. The time he went to elaborate lengths to convince his kids that pasta grows on trees. The time he was working in Kuwait, and the hotel chef was so terrible that after a day laying cables and installing TVs, David would knock up dinner for the guests of the entire hotel.

When they come out to the graveside, the rain has stopped. David's daughter sings a beautiful, uplifting song. Then the celebrant says it's time to say farewell to David. '*At the salting of our food we remember him...At the squeaking of a dog ball we remember him...*' There's a trug full of petals for people to throw onto the grave. (Someone asks later, 'That was so lovely, where did you get those from?' and Louisa says 'I ripped the heads off roses. Someone went to Tesco's and we ripped the heads off.' It seemed appropriate at the time.) As they slowly lower the coffin and throw the rose petals, the sun comes out and everyone's saying, 'David's done this!' Louisa doesn't literally believe that, but he was such an optimist that it feels right and normal for the sun to shine.

The kids have put six big collage boards with pictures of David around the pub. His grinning face. One of the staff says, would you like tea or coffee, or Prosecco? 'Prosecco!' they all say, 'We want Prosecco!' Obviously. Everyone stands round drinking and laughing and at one point you think, *where's David?* Because the only thing missing from this gathering of all his friends is him. The love – and this sounds hippy-dippy – but the love in the room is palpable. There's more to us than surgeons can take apart. It isn't religion and it isn't God, Louisa's sure of that. It is to do with people being together, making each other feel better.

If death is a test of people's commitment and love, it could not have been more underlined in David's case. They're a hotchpotch of step relations and exes. It was not until the funeral and the aftermath that Louisa knew the depths of how *family* they were. She has fantastic support around her. But she misses him. The man she loved is never coming back. Louisa doesn't know why it should be such a shock. She knew he was dying. He knew he was dying. He smoked for 50 years and you know no good can come of that. Why is she so surprised somehow? Maybe she is just sad. David was a Churchill man. There's that quote – 'If you're going through hell, keep going.' And what else can you do?

David had emphysema, from smoking, and sarcoidosis, an industrial disease they think he might have acquired 20 years back. Because his lung capacity was so small, he got heart failure and you can't live forever with that. His businesses were up and down, he no longer owned property. But he wanted to make sure the kids would have a little something. He had term insurance, a policy that would pay out if he died within ten years. He kept saying in the last few years, 'The kids will be alright, they'll be alright.' David and Louisa would say to each other 'We ought to get our ducks in a row.' They both re-wrote their wills, he made her a director of his businesses, wrote down all – well, most – of his passwords. You've got to get your ducks in a row. And all the time, they'd both be thinking *enough about the fucking ducks.* But now she is exceptionally grateful for all David did to smooth out some of those practicalities. He died 18 months or so within that ten-year term, so he did manage to line a couple of those ducks up.

His health was in a downward trajectory those last two years. But it was so incremental, such a small chipping away, you sort of didn't notice. When

David died, a lot of people said, 'Oh God, I didn't realise he was so ill.' Louisa said to them, 'Don't you remember, when we came round to your house he was on bottled oxygen?' 'Oh, I don't remember that.' Because he played it down. When people asked him how he was, he'd say 'Oh, I'm fine.' There's not a point where you go from not being disabled to being disabled. It was a very slow thing. Louisa would take the dog out when they couldn't do it together any more. Then she would be the one to hump the shopping from the car. But David could put a positive spin on absolutely anything. When he had to use the mobility scooter to get about, he didn't complain, he said, 'Oh, I can go out now.' Everything was 'Look what I'm able to do now because I'm on this medication, or I've seen this doctor.' When he got his blue badge, he could *officially* drive up to anywhere and park outside. He was living, he wasn't dying. A month before he died, he said, 'Everyone's telling me this has been a shit year, but it hasn't really.' His son had got a lovely girlfriend. His daughter and Louisa's were both at university doing 'proper degrees.' The other daughter was forging a good career and had just got engaged. He and Louisa had got married. He said, 'I can't say I've had a bad year. I'm happy.'

The other thing about really knowing death is coming, is you get more of a 'Yeah, fuck it!' attitude. The two of them were very much, 'Shall we do that? Let's.' They went on honeymoon in September and the car broke down, so they didn't get to do everything they wanted. In November he said, 'Let's go on honeymoon again then.' And they did. By that time David was really quite ill, but they had a couple of nights in a hotel in Norfolk. And they got to celebrate New Year's Eve. Neither of them could quite believe he was still alive. *Wow! Into another year!* It felt like extra time. These days, Louisa has found herself crawling round the North Circular to the office, and she'll think, *if I die tomorrow, is this what I want to have been doing?* She knows now, life's too short. So she'll change her plan, call in, do something else, or perhaps just go home.

David is buried at a place called Sun Rising. It's not the nearest natural burial ground, but it's the one that felt right, and it's dog-friendly. Once it's full, it will carry on being run as a nature reserve. Louisa went up there in May, when all the lace-white cow parsley was out. The dog pissed a few times – David would have loved that! It's nice to have a place to go to. It's not like he resides there. But they planted an oak tree to mark the actual spot and it feels nice to think of it growing there. The atoms that make you don't disappear. If you're buried, the stuff that makes you goes into the ground and some of that stuff gets re-formed into other living things. It's not as if David's suddenly become a tree, but bits of him are there.

When people have a kid together, the whole becomes greater than the sum of its parts. You actually make another person. Louisa and David didn't make another person. Those days were behind them when they met. They had a dog instead, their baby. With tight black curls and a thumping tail. Holidays, their wedding – everything had to include the dog. And now Louisa's life is geared around the dog, which pisses her off rather, because it's like being a single parent again and he won't grow up and go to university, because he's not *that* clever. She worries about losing him, though, because he does feel like part of David. He'd had lots of dogs before, but Harris was probably his favourite. She has the dog to thank for staying sane. What can sometimes be sad about not having religion is not being part of a community. Having a dog, though, you're part of this other world, you belong to something. When you're out in the park with a dog, people talk to you. Louisa takes Harris out at seven every morning. There will be half a dozen other people out, sometimes more. People whose lives would never otherwise cross. There's a cake-maker, a choreographer, and a therapist; a dog-minder, a hairdresser, and a fellow recent-widow; a London tour guide, a nurse, and two people whose jobs Louisa doesn't understand. They never would have met if it weren't for the dogs, but now Louisa knows about their family weddings, what their kids are studying, the places they've been. She could loaf in bed and walk the dog later, but she'll be up and out because she doesn't want to miss those little interactions.

Another new bit of life that's come to Louisa from David's death is the volunteering that she does now. David had volunteered with Contact the Elderly for years, ferrying mostly old ladies to tea parties once a month. When he got too ill to drive, he didn't want to give it up, so Louisa came with him. It got a tad bizarre – towards the end, the Elderly were fitter than David by far – and the Christmas party was particularly absurd. David and Louisa were in charge of leading Christmas carols, though they were both Jewish by birth and didn't really know the words. Harris was terrified by the bangs of Christmas crackers. So, you've got a hysterical dog that's desperate to get out, and a man on oxygen in a jaunty party hat!

After David died, Louisa didn't want to do the ferrying round, but she volunteered to be one of their tea party hosts. The ladies came one July day and it felt like a positive thing, and they sent lovely thank you cards with squiggly handwriting. It is not quite that she is continuing *for* him, more that it's a good thing to do and she wasn't quite a good enough person to do it before she met him. She bought a bun not long after he died but didn't have the appetite to eat it. Instead of putting it in the bin, she gave it to a homeless person. She wouldn't have done that, before knowing David. He was a sucker for giving people stuff. He'd turn out his pockets.

You had to be careful when at the shops with David, because if you said, 'I really like that,' he'd buy it for you. Coming up to that last Christmas, he intimated Louisa would be getting a new duvet (*how unromantic*, she thought). What he presented her with on the morning – because she'd happened to say how nice it was in a shop a few weeks earlier – was a swan. Not a painting or model, but a full size, real, stuffed, massive swan. Wings spread, as if about to take off from its plinth. She looks at it now and thinks that man was a lesson in how to be happy – and she can keep on learning from him.

*

When Louisa responded to my request to speak to non-religious people about happiness at the end of life, it had been just two weeks since David's death. I worried it might be too soon for her to tell me about what they'd been through together and what she, now, was going through without him. She replied asking what difference it would make to wait a little longer – since the man she loved was never coming back. That pain wasn't about to go away. When Louisa lost David, she lost the person with whom she'd been most intimately connected; the person who'd been by her side was gone. As things turned out, by the time we met, eight months had passed since David's death. Louisa told me how she'd got through those first months. Though there was never any possibility of filling that David-shaped hole, she expressed her deep appreciation for those who'd come closer to her following his death. They helped her carry her pain and take steps forward. She has learned that 'family' love can extend beyond blood ties; been warmed by the 'group hug' of those remembering David on Facebook; and found a comforting sense of community amongst fellow dog-walkers. For Louisa, as for many others who shared their stories with me, the day of her loved one's funeral offered a treasured sense of connection and support through her early days of grief.

12

MARGARET

and non-religious funerals

As a nation, we are no longer satisfied with the kind of funeral where someone stands and talks about what they think happens in a world beyond, and not about the person we have lost. In 2019, a report published by Co-operative Funeralcare, the UK's largest provider of funerals, noted that over a quarter (27%) of British adults would want an entirely non-religious funeral service, whilst just 10% of people said that they would want a traditional religious funeral. Over three quarters of Co-op's funeral directors have noticed an increase in requests for funerals to take place outside of traditional religious settings; and more families are requesting that a celebrant – rather than a religious leader – conduct their loved one's funeral.

As Louisa experienced, a funeral free from religious content, which focuses on celebrating the unique life of our lost loved one, can be a great comfort. The tribute offers an opportunity to piece together all the little quirks, those milestone moments, along with anecdotes from various sources, to form a picture of a whole person. A funeral brings people together to collectively reminisce and cherish the person who has died, and to support each other. It is a day on which we acknowledge both that death is real, and that life is precious. Most people, in planning a loved one's funeral, aim for a ceremony which reflects the beliefs and values of the person who has died. A funeral ceremony that feels right – like a fitting way to honour our loved one – can be an important early step towards healing, towards rediscovering a sense of hope and meaning in our lives. Many non-religious people choose a humanist funeral ceremony.

*

At the Roman Catholic funeral service for Margaret's father, what she heard was platitudes and lies, the standard hymns, the usual prayers, and very little about the dad she knew. At the first humanist funeral Margaret went to, though, there was no mention of ashes or dust. There was laughter and joy and it was all about Sheila, Margaret's friend who had died. Margaret thought, everyone deserves a send-off like that, and she decided to train as a humanist celebrant herself, attracted by the value humanism places on living this one life with honesty and kindness.

When she visits a family, one of the first things she'll tell them is 'From the time you arrive at the crematorium till the time you leave, I will be personally responsible for everything. I will look after you and you don't need to worry.' They will sigh and say, 'Oh that's really good.' And they will begin to feel supported. Margaret stays with the family for around two hours; she shows them she's a human being and tries to create a space of trust where they can say whatever they want to say. If the family have been caring for someone who had dementia, she may say 'That must have been really difficult, you must have been really tired,' and perhaps even 'You must have found it difficult to like them sometimes.' She tries to allow people to own their anger, or resentment, or whatever feelings they may have which otherwise they'd feel guilty about. She may say to people, 'Whatever you feel now, it's ok for you to feel,' because sometimes people need that permission.

Last week, Margaret was with a woman, Penny, whose husband George had died suddenly at the wheel with her in the passenger seat. Margaret said 'How shocking! How terrible for you! I can't imagine how I'd feel if that happened to me,' and that allowed Penny to say 'It was so awful, Margaret, I thought I was going to die.' When Margaret arrived, Penny and her three children were distraught, but by the time she left they were laughing together. How is that possible? It happens when you acknowledge the death, the great loss, but also remember that this was a whole, living person. You let the family talk about the person they loved and show you photographs. It will be things like – 'What was he like as a husband? Did he buy you birthday cards? Did he cook for you? What made him special?' She'll ask about what mattered to that person, and she'll stay with the family until she's discovered what she thinks is the essence of the person who has died. 'Tell me, what did he like doing, was he a good gardener, was he good at DIY?' 'No, he was useless at it!' The laughter is so healing. After the family visit, Margaret will put the ceremony together, and she'll share iterations of the tribute until the family are comfortable with it, so that there are no surprises on the day.

During the service, Margaret will reflect that death is hard and that no religion or philosophy can prevent sorrow as a natural reaction to the loss of a loved one. She may say something like 'Grief is a reflection of our love, and yes there will be tears today, but I hope there will be smiles, even a little laughter as we recall a unique man. We intend today to be about the gift of Jim and not about his loss.' Sometimes she'll quote the words of the Greek statesman Pericles, 'What you leave behind is not what is engraved in stone monuments, but what is woven into the lives of others.' There will be readings chosen by the family, and often it will be the same few choices. Words such as 'An afterglow of smiles when life is done,' or 'It was beautiful/As long as it lasted/The journey of my life.' The most popular funeral poem of all is 'He is gone': 'You can shed tears because he is gone/Or you can smile because he has lived.' Margaret has done 'He is gone' or 'She is gone' maybe 600 times. Clichéd words are clichés for a reason - because they work for people, and contain some fundamental truths. Most of the service, though, will be given over to words about the life and legacy of the particular person who has died. In a religious funeral, if the assumption is that someone has gone onto another life, and you want to recognise that, then that religious content takes up time; in traditional crematoria, time is limited, so if you've got to get in that stuff about a life to come, it reduces the amount of time you have to talk about the life that person has lived. In preparing the tribute, Margaret tries to pull together a complete picture of the person from what family and friends have said, and if she's done it well, people will come up to her afterwards and say, 'It was as if you'd known Joyce all your life.' She can give those left behind the gift of knowing bits of their loved one they never knew before – allow grandchildren to see a frail lady as she was at 20, beautiful and vital. The family receives printed copies of the tribute, and sometimes she'll get emails months down the line, saying 'I've just read your tribute again, and it made me smile.'

Margaret believes what gives a funeral value for the ones left behind, is honesty, authenticity. She once did a funeral for a murderer, and she didn't say 'He was a good man,' because he wasn't. He'd been very damaged and he'd hurt lots of people, and just saying that allowed people to feel we're allowed to be angry and upset. She doesn't try to pretend that everything's ok when it is not. She said, 'What he did caused so much harm, but the one good thing that has come out of it is that this trauma has brought people together.' If it's a child who has died, you can't say 'Their time has come;' you have to acknowledge how horrible it is, how wrong. This shouldn't be about death now, this should be about life and looking forward to the future. And even so, you have to try to find something positive, some glimmer of hope at a very dark time. Margaret was celebrant at a funeral for a baby who lived only a day, and she said, 'Look at us, how we've all been drawn together here, how everyone is supporting everyone else and saying things we never would normally, about how much we love and care for each other.' You draw out the positives for people to hold onto. You can't take away the pain, but you can maybe soften it a little bit.

Last month, Margaret did the funeral for her friend Isobel, who had died aged 57. She thought I can do this, but when she saw the coffin she almost lost it for a moment – thinking my friend's in that box. It mattered, though, that she held it together for the family's sake. Her voice cracked a couple of times during the service, but that was ok, because people were aware she knew and cared for Isobel. Mostly, she is able to put some kind of emotional barrier up, but there is a cumulative effect. She puts love into what she does, and she tries to walk a little way with each family on their journey. Sometimes she feels she's like a sponge soaking up the family's feelings; she gets rid of some of that on paper when she writes the ceremony, but she's left with some residual sorrow, grief, anger, and she is conscious that the time is coming for her to say goodbye to celebrancy. It's time now for Margaret to move on to a new chapter; she feels satisfaction closing this one, knowing she's helped 760 bereaved families begin to say goodbye, in a way that felt fitting for their loved ones and for them.

*

I spoke to Margaret on the phone; we never met in person. Her warmth, compassion and authenticity came through strongly as she spoke. When I die, I hope someone like Margaret speaks about me.

13

MARIAM AND ZAHEER

when the funeral doesn't fit

It's a good thing that more and more UK funerals, like Margaret's humanist ceremonies, now allow scope for a personalised celebration of the individual who has died. Unfortunately, though, it remains fairly common for non-religious grievers to have to sit through a funeral that feels wrong for them and may also fail to reflect the world view of their loved one. When a funeral does not feel fitting, it cannot be a step towards healing, but instead may add to the trauma of loss, as was the case for Mariam.

*

When Mariam's brother died in his twenties, she told her parents 'You *cannot* bury my brother – he wanted to be cremated, he didn't want a Muslim burial.' They knew this – they knew their son was atheist, that he thought religion was 'all bollocks.' But it was always about what *they* believed, and it was always about saving face in the community, and so he had a Muslim burial. In the mosque, Mariam longed to go to her brother, but was told 'A woman should not touch a man's dead body.' Many members of the extended family had shown up, people who'd never been there for her brother while he was still alive. Mariam had nothing to say to these people. When she saw several of her brother's friends, though, she wanted to support them, cuddle and console them. (The following day, her parents received a phone call from a family member saying, 'Mariam was hugging white men at her brother's funeral – she should have more shame.') One of his female friends was wearing a black skirt – it was just above the knee, perhaps; the family stared at her with disgust. Mariam told her, 'Just ignore them. You're here for my brother – he loved you and you loved him, simple.' Mariam's partner, Ollie, wasn't at the funeral. That morning, her mum had said, 'He can come so long as he tells no one who he is, goes nowhere near you, doesn't touch you.' Of course, those were impossible conditions.

Afterwards, though, he was there for her. And like a lot of ex-Muslim girls who've been ostracised from their communities, Mariam has made her own family. Ollie's family have welcomed her; she's lucky, too, in the close friends she has made whom she knows are always there for her. Some people say they can count their good friends on one hand; Mariam would need three hands to count hers. The people who love her get that if she doesn't want to talk, there's nothing coming out; they let it all be on her terms. They get that sometimes she'll just want to watch crap tv, eat something nice. At first, it was very hard for Mariam to take on board that her brother wanted her to go on, to have a good life with Ollie. Some days are very hard, still, but now she tries to remember her brother's hopes for her, focuses on what can still be good and happy.

Like Mariam, Zaheer was unable to find comfort in the Muslim funeral held for his loved one. In this case, the ceremony did reflect his mother's religious world view, but for Zaheer, an agnostic, the service held no meaning. As the prescribed prayers and rituals were carried out, he was sat there thinking, *she's gone now, what difference does it make what you say and don't say and the order that you say it in?* There was something for him, though, in the Muslim practice of observing a three-day period of mourning following the funeral. A stream of visitors came to the family home to pay their respects, say prayers, bring food. There was a warmth in being surrounded by people who cared about his mum, even though he didn't share their religious beliefs.

His mum had died aged 65 following complications after kidney transplant surgery. She'd been ill for a long time with diabetes that led to kidney failure, but her death still felt sudden and unexpected. Before the transplant, she'd been going downhill, and began to talk of her acceptance of death. She felt that she was halfway there, and that didn't seem to frighten her; she believed Allah would decide when her time came. But when her chance for a transplant came up, she never thought she wouldn't make it through and neither did Zaheer. She was just so elated about getting the kidney. When she died, Zaheer struggled to make sense of it at first; he was looking for some kind of explanation. Over time, he had to accept that her heart had simply been too weak to withstand the strain of surgery. After the three-day mourning period had ended, things got a bit quiet. There was a big hole in his life because he had been close to his mum and had been used to seeing her on a weekly basis when he took her for dialysis, or sometimes for a shopping trip. He didn't know what to do with that quiet and that hole. But he has a supportive girlfriend, who is there and listens. And he has old friends to have a beer with. Now that both parents have gone, he has a sense of being next in line, as if somehow his mum and dad had been standing between him and death. His growing awareness that time is limited pushes Zaheer to go out and do things, to go for a run or bike ride: he thinks of how inactive his parents became as they got older, and how that didn't help them. That awareness of how short time is also pushes him to connect, make plans with friends more often, to meet and laugh and chat.

*

I've tended to ask those sharing their stories with me whether they ever *wish* they could believe in an afterlife, or that everything happens as it is meant to. Some have answered yes to one or both of these questions. Zaheer, though unable to live by the Muslim faith his parents had tried to instil in him, told me that for him the idea of a heaven remained more appealing than the thought that everything just stops. Some who've lost a religious faith mourn that loss; though the evidence of the world pushes them to let go of their religious beliefs, it may be harder to let go of the wishing-it-were-so.

Yet when Arthur first contacted me, he told me that 'strange as this may seem to believers,' he and his wife, Wendy, both felt their non-religious life stance had helped them to cope with loss.

14

ARTHUR

in our life there is a single colour

It is coming up to seven years since Arthur and Wendy's only son Ian died from T-cell lymphoma, five months short of his 30th birthday. This is what they now call 'The Biggie.' The one big sadness in their otherwise happy lives together.

Arthur has never had any anger, for which he is grateful. Anger can be such a destructive emotion. If he believed in God, he would never have forgiven Him/Her/It. In the early days he used to tell people that on the infinitesimally small, 0.000000000001% chance that there is a God, and Arthur ever met Him, he would call Him a bastard and spit in His eye, for cutting Ian's life short, for not making the treatment work, not answering the prayers offered up by religious friends. But as things are, it has always helped Arthur and Wendy not to have to torture themselves wondering *why us?* There's no reason for such things, other than bad luck.

As for Ian's beliefs – for the hospital admission notes, when asked his religion Ian told them 'Heavy Metal.' He later discovered on the form at the bottom of his bed, they had recorded 'none', and asked for that to be corrected. He really felt that the bands he loved gave him power in his heart when times were hard, just as others may turn to their faith. He'd have been chuffed to know that in the national census the year after he died, 6,242 folk recorded themselves as sharing his heavy metal religion.

Ian was diagnosed in the February, and from then, until his death on December 15th, Arthur and Wendy were with him virtually every day. When your children are at school, you don't see them that much, just at the end of the day. When they're teenagers, they do their own thing. Then they get a job and move away from home. In that last year, they were more involved with Ian's daily life than they had been since he was very small, spent more time together than some parents get with their kids in a lifetime. In some ways it was a special year.

He had six lots of chemo, of the kind you had to have as a hospital inpatient. And then if he got an infection while his body was immunosuppressed, he'd have to be kept in longer than the usual week. During that year, Ian had to spend about 100 days in hospital. On one of those days, Ian said to his dad, 'This is shit, but some folk have worse shit to put up with all their lives. We have great lives normally and this is just temporary, so we'll get through it.' That was something Arthur noted down in his little cork-bound book of truths and uplifting thoughts. Ian had worked with adults with severe mental and physical disabilities, so he knew about the struggles people face. In Ian's diary for that year, the days in hospital are left blank. But when he came out, he'd class each as 'a good day/a shit day/ a great day.' There were still, in that cancer year, about 45 great days. Mostly, they were good or ok days, and only a few – while he was out of hospital – were classed as shit. Wendy wasn't so sure they should read his diary – it was Ian's – and Arthur doesn't read it often. But at the time, adding up the days like that was some help. To know that life for Ian in his last year was mostly still good, or even great.

And before that last year, Ian had many years of going to gigs, travelling, various jobs, two girlfriends. He knew the pleasures of sex and being in love and the heartaches of breaking up. He'd experienced quite a bit of life. He'd grown tall enough to dwarf both his parents, to pat them on their heads.

Ian was working in Switzerland when he first landed in hospital for investigation. He was told he had a lesion at the base of his spine. It was a shock to him to find out later that meant cancer. Wendy and Arthur flew out to be with him for the operation and afterwards the three of them came home together. After the diagnosis, Ian wanted to have a Living Will. So it's 'Do you want life-extending treatment in such and such circumstances, or do you want drugs that will keep you out of pain, even if it's at the risk of shortening your life?' Ian wrote that he wanted the pain relief. He knew it might come to that. They knew it was a bad cancer, but there was a treatment, so that was it, they just tried to get their heads round 'Right, we're going for the cure.' Arthur is a biologist by background, so he could have looked stuff up on the internet, and he did a bit in the beginning, but Ian didn't want to hear about it, so Arthur never researched in great detail after that. They all just hoped the stem treatment and the BEAM chemotherapy was going to do it. It was Wendy's idea to call themselves the 'E-Team', from the first letter of their surname and inspired by a certain popular '80s show. They were the E-Team, in it together! They'd go into a trio hug. Arthur still has a text message from a time Ian needed a transfusion – 'Hi my bestest plumpies, I've just started on my 3rd bag of blood so come and get me as soon as you can please. Love you loads.'

There was only the one time…and this was after a lot of chemo, after the prognosis was down from 50-50 to about 20%, and they were having to wait around for yet another test. The two of them were alone in a hospital room and Ian said to his dad, 'How would you cope? How will you and Mum cope, if I do die, without me?' Then there were weepy hugs. And when Arthur could get out an answer, it was, 'I haven't a clue, son. It will crucify us. But we'll still have each other… *But,*' he told his son, 'we're not there yet. You're young, you're strong, why can't you be one of the 20%?' and Ian seemed to accept that. Macmillan are right when they say 'living with cancer is still living.' It has to be. You get on with it and try not to dwell on your fears. So it was, 'Let's enjoy, as soon as we're out of hospital.' They got away that weekend, to Cambridge and it wasn't one of the greatest holidays ever, but they had as good a Saturday and Sunday as they could.

Soon after that, during a stay in hospital, Ian made a list of places where he wanted his ashes scattered if it came to that. And another list, four sides of names of friends to whom he assigned specific items from his music collection. He recorded messages to be played at his funeral, to introduce his favourite metal tracks. It all seemed relatively easy because it was just an insurance policy in case the worst happened. And who really believes they'll need insurance when they take it out? He'd amuse the nurses with visions of mourners all in football shirts, of older relatives headbanging to thrash metal. How can death be real in the mind of a 28, 29-year-old young man?

Ian died on the 15th December, but, for Arthur, it is from the 5th each year that the sadness and foreboding will tend to build up. That is the date on which they – though not Ian – were told there was no longer any hope. They were back in hospital. The chemo drugs had affected Ian's kidneys and he became delirious. It was hard for Arthur and Wendy, but Ian didn't really know what was going on, he just kept cussing Man United. (He was a Liverpool FC man.) That's when the doctor told Arthur and Wendy that the treatment hadn't worked, the cancer cells were still there, and there was no more powerful treatment they could give him. Arthur said 'Please don't tell Ian. It's bad enough for him already, and I don't know how he'd cope, knowing he's definitely going to die.' The doctor said, 'If he asks, we'll have to tell him.' They put Ian on more fluids and he became coherent again for a few days. The three of them played simple card games. Ian was able to talk to other people in the ward, and even said to a lady visiting someone else, 'Oh give us a hug!' which she did, and when she asked how Ian was doing, he said that he'd had the stem cell transplant and you just had to hope and stay positive. One of the staff even said, 'It's a big improvement isn't it?' Arthur and Wendy thought *well, no, it isn't really*. It was only a temporary respite. But Ian never asked any questions, 'How am I doing?' or 'What's going to happen?' so he was never told his death was inevitable.

Then one day he suddenly had shooting pains, and because he'd signed a Living Will to say he didn't want to suffer unnecessarily, the head of the ward was brilliant, he got a morphine pump ready and within five minutes from being in foot-stamping, clenching pain, Ian was unconscious, peaceful. He died five days later without ever really becoming fully awake. Arthur and Wendy can't know all that went through Ian's mind towards the end, but they think their son never knew he was definitely going to die. That's one of the things, looking back, that helps them cope. And apart from those five foot-stamping minutes, there wasn't disastrous suffering, which was something.

It was difficult, after Ian died, for Arthur and Wendy to see any purpose left in their lives. They'd been retired for around eight years, all four of their parents had died, and now their only child had gone. What was there left to live for? For the last year, they'd been with Ian almost every day. Now he was gone, what did they have? A void. A gaping hole.

The two of them went away for a week once Ian's funeral was over, and Arthur came up with 'I suppose we'll just have to start making new memories for ourselves,' which Wendy said really helped her. The following year, they bought a small second-hand motorhome, which they try to get away in at least one weekend a month.

It was Arthur's idea to set up the trust in Ian's name. Wendy wasn't sure, but she eventually agreed, on the understanding they would do it for five years. She didn't want the charity to take over their lives, and running it could not bring Ian back. Which of course is what they'd want most in the world. Arthur wanted to feel he was doing something, that something good could come from Ian's passing. He was grateful that in that last year, they had been able to get away in between rounds of treatment, sometimes at less than 24 hours' notice. They couldn't go too far – they'd have to rush Ian back to hospital if his temperature rose – but they saw some beautiful parts of the UK. Short walks in the countryside. Meals and real ales in the local CAMRA-recommended pubs. These were the days which made that year bearable. These are the days that still give Arthur and Wendy joy, looking back. The day they revisited a favourite Lakes valley, where Ian had volunteered six years earlier, rebuilding a wall that runs up the fell. The day they went walking by the South Stack cliffs and lighthouse at Anglesey, watching seabirds on the wing. They were financially secure enough not to have to worry too much about the cost of holiday accommodation, which isn't true for everyone. The trust in Ian's name was set up to help others whose lives had been turned upside down by a blood cancer. It would give those in financial need the chance to take a break during a brief interval between their spells of intensive treatment.

Fundraising brings a new impetus – you try things you would not otherwise have done. Climb a mountain. Run a marathon. Fundraising events bring people together. To see one of Ian's mates getting a cake to the face for sponsorship. To see Arthur getting drenched by a bucket of ice-cold water. Ian had expressed his passion for metal music and for football through collecting memorabilia. Arthur sold his metal t-shirts and football shirts on eBay to raise money for the trust. One of the best sellers was a child's sky-blue Sunderland away shirt from the 1990s, which went for £75. It was nice to think the shirt would now be special to someone else.

All told, the trust raised £57,414, and helped over 250 oncology patients to enjoy morale-boosting day trips and short breaks. Much of the money was distributed at three local hospitals by social workers, who told Arthur of the joy it gifted patients in the planning, the anticipation, and the experience itself of time away from Cancerland. Arthur heard of one young girl with bone cancer, admitted for the amputation of her leg, and how the prospect of a short break in the Lake District brought a smile to her face in the midst of tears.

They donated Ian's fussball table to a local children's ward, where it was installed in their spacious new rec room. Arthur and Wendy spent an hour putting all the rods of players back into position again. The ward caters for young people between 11 and 18, suffering from a variety of blood and bone cancers, many of whom have trouble walking, but who can stand and twiddle knobs just fine. Perhaps, at this very moment, that little ball is pinging in the goal.

Arthur spent a pleasant morning pinning Ian's collection of Liverpool badges onto two large England flags. He thinks Ian would have liked to see them all arranged that way, only he was so busy collecting he never got around to displaying them together. It was a satisfying moment to stand back and see something completed. It gives Arthur a smile one day when, having a clear out, he finds a diary from when Ian was 19 – "Did the usual jobs and on my break decided to play keep-ups on the lawn. Beat my previous record of 88 and got to 150 – Yeeeeeesssss! However, this did make me sweaty and not a nice person to be around, but what the hell – 150!"

Arthur and Wendy, along with some of Ian's friends, scattered or buried Ian's ashes according to his wishes in several places that were meaningful to him. The one they return to sometimes, is a bit of woodland in Leicestershire with a view over a reservoir. A good path goes around it, giving a pleasant three-mile stroll. Initially they left the spot unmarked, but when they discovered a bench with a memorial to another person alongside Ian's ashes, they felt they should do something to let folk know the place was important to other people too, so they put a small plaque in. They visit once a year or so, to keep the area clear of brambles and ivy, and it's nice to see signs that others have been joining in that effort. They raise a toast in Ian's memory when they go. One of his precious brews – Sink the Bismarck, Jaipur IPA, or Tokyo oak-aged stout.

So, now it is coming up to the seventh anniversary of Ian's death. Arthur and Wendy will spend some time talking, looking over things. One may need to correct the odd detail from the other's memory of something. This is important because it is in their memories that Ian lives now. They'll look over photographs and the DVD of the 'Celebration of Ian's Life.' From the opening sequences, it makes Arthur smile at what they managed to put together based on Ian's choice of music. Medieval metal can be quite nice really, but they did have to warn some of Ian's older relatives to bring earplugs for the more snarly, thrash metal selections. Arthur speaks of his best football buddy, and of standing side by side with Ian at a match back in September. As they sang 'You'll Never Walk Alone,' Arthur tried not to let his son see on his face the tears of fear that this would be their last time here together. In the order of service they've added a note – 'or in Ian's case "You Never Walked Alone"' – and it is good to see how true that is. So many of Ian's friends have come together to celebrate him and now they sing loud in his honour, football scarves raised and swaying above their heads. 'Walk on, walk on, with hope in your heart.' The whole event is peppered with all the classic Ian-isms. Arthur says he'll miss the amusingly-rude shape into which Ian would peel a satsuma skin – and holds one up for demonstration purposes... The celebrant reads out a post from his

MySpace page: 'I like epic soaring fast bands that make me want to oil myself up, put on a loin cloth, grab my sword and run up a mountain to shout from the top… Sadly this has only happened in my bedroom.' And then you hear Ian's own recorded voice: 'Thank you all very much for coming to my funeral.' He hopes it's been a celebration, rather than a negative experience. 'Now it's time to leave, and what better way to get you to bugger off quickly than a track by Rotting Christ?'

Arthur recently became aware of an opportunity to have Ian's name memorialised on a stone at Anfield, and he decided to splash out. He realises now what he's been doing these last seven years – finding ways to get Ian mentioned as permanently as he can. He is trying to ensure that Ian's relatively short time on earth means something; 29 years was not enough really for him to make much of a mark himself, though he did more in his decade or so as a young man than many others do. And, of course, his many, many mates will remember him until they die. Arthur still remembers one of his close mates who died back in the 70s, so he knows 100% that Ian's mates will remember him, always. One of them has even had a tattoo in Ian's honour. Though Ian was a MySpace man and never was on Facebook, within days of his death, two Facebook tribute pages had sprung up, where many expressed what Ian meant to them: 'a top bloke,' 'always there for me,' 'Ian always made a night out better.'

It was on one of these nights out with his mates, after a few beers, that the idea of a CAMRA equivalent for cheese was floated, and so CHURCH was born: the Campaign Honouring Unique Real CHeese. The likes of Dairylea and Babybel would not be welcome. The likes of St Nectaire and Veritable Chaumes, however, would be consumed with gusto. One summer evening in a pub garden somewhere, Ian stood up on a picnic table and recited his 'ode to cheese.' All present were duly inaugurated into CHURCH, in the name of Cheesus, amen. Ian's mates will remember him. It's the generations to come, the future family genealogists, who maybe aren't yet born, that Arthur's trying to put a sign out to with the Anfield stone, the plaque next to his ashes, the funeral transcript lodged in the Bishopsgate Institute archives. They are ways he tries to help Ian reach out into the future – proof that he existed that will survive his parents' deaths.

Arthur and Wendy will never experience the joy and consolation of grandchildren. Arthur's niece, Emma, will still have around 25% of his genes, her children 12.5% and so on. But for any of us, 20, 50 generations on, our descendants will have only a tiny fraction of our genes. It is weirdly comforting to Arthur that we're all just part of a huge human gene pool! One anniversary, a neighbour sent a card quoting the artist Marc Chagall –

'In our life there is a single colour, as on an artist's palette, which provides the meaning of life and art. It is the colour of love.' Arthur thought, *yes, that's all that really matters. For other creatures, it's the urge to reproduce, for us it's love. A couple could have 10-20 grandchildren, but that would mean little if there were no deep love there.* The two surviving members of the E-team have that deep love, no question, brought even closer – if that were possible – by their loss.

On the anniversary this year, Arthur shares with Wendy his re-discovered diary from the summer he retired, when Ian was 22. The last entry reads 'Bad night's kip – stayed up until 1am but Ian still not in and he eventually came in very drunk and zombie-ish at 3.30am and then sat on the loo asleep until almost 5am when I managed to get some water into him and into bed.' The joys and worries of parenthood! So there is that. They don't have to worry about him any more. They will never have to see him growing old. And unlike many of their friends and neighbours, Arthur and Wendy's retirement is unencumbered by child care. They are free to set off in their motorhome making new memories for themselves. Ian never set foot in the van of course, yet in a way he's there with them. He had bought some melamine ware with a cheerful orange Gazania flower design, intended as a present to his parents for the Christmas that he never saw. As soon as they bought the motorhome, the plates and bowls went straight in and their food goes on those orange flowers every breakfast, every evening, every trip. It means a lot to have that gift from Ian with them; their new memories are coloured by his love.

15

BOB

and his search for meaning in a living place

It is a Friday afternoon, so here he is. Bob's a busy bloke otherwise, rushing around all week, but on a Friday afternoon he'll be here, on Vera's south-facing bench. If he's got something complicated to think about, then sitting here, seeing the clouds moving, tends to help. He talks to her sometimes, if he feels like it, tells her what's going on. If he has family phone calls to make, he makes them here, so that in some way, Vera is included. Last week the leaves of her tree were still tight in the bud; today they have unfurled. Every time he comes, something is different. It's a living place. Vera's beech tree is ten years old now, and around 16 feet tall. The flowers around her spot are ones that Bob and Vera used to go and look for when they first married. Vera was the one who knew more about wildflowers; Bob has learnt a lot more about them since she died, so that he could track them down and get them here for her. When the Viper's Bugloss comes up in a few weeks, its flowers first pink, then shading to intense ultramarine, it will take him back to the cliffs above Beer Head in Cornwall, where they sat one afternoon in their early days, she sewing something, he reading a book.

He tends to put new plug plants in each spring, but by now the place has its own rotation going – the snowdrops start, then come the primroses, the cowslips. He knows when he's under the ground with her, the flowers will carry on, and that's good, that's what he wants to see, really. He sends photos round as the seasons change, so the family – his three sons, their wives and kids – can keep in touch with the flowers. They'll say, 'That's nice, what's that one?' and so on. There is no marker on the grave itself – only the flowers show its approximate location. In the winter months, the

76

edges of the excavation are still discernible, but it makes Bob very happy to see that the wildflower seeds now have spread beyond the vicinity of Vera's grave. Right now, he's got the bluebells for company, and a light breeze moving through.

Vera died ten years ago, 60 years young, from lung cancer and a brain tumour. Bob and Vera chose this cemetery even before she got ill. In her last ten years, she'd got into family history. She and Bob happened to come here looking for her ancestors' graves. They picked up a leaflet about woodland burial and decided that's what they wanted. For the most part, this place is a standard cemetery, but in the corner acre where she's buried, there's this long grass, graves amongst trees. They liked the idea, because a tree puts something back, not like a dead granite gravestone, imported from China – think of the carbon miles in that lot! Bob's grandparents' graves are those old concrete jobs, they just deteriorate, it's bloody awful. And if the gravestones are to be kept neat, the grass needs cutting every week, and strimming round them – all that fuel… But with this acre of young trees, it's twice a year the grass gets cut, that's it. The cemetery staff all know him, as he's been going so often and for so long. A few years back the manager said 'Bob, that woodland area looks like it's just rough grass and people let their dogs run over it because they don't know. How can we show it's a special area but still part of the cemetery?' Bob said he thought a post and rail fence, so they put one in, and that's made a difference. It used to be, with woodland burial, each grave had its own tree. Of course, space runs out eventually. Bob's booked to go in next to her, and the two of them can share the tree; he wouldn't want them digging round the roots of Vera's beech to put another in, with risk of causing damage.

Bob's parents were both cremated, as they wanted, down at Eastbourne, and he visits once a year, but there's nowhere to visit really, they were scattered. With Vera it's different, this is her bit, and he does feel close to her here. He is faithful in his visits, though he has no faith. If he sits quietly and lets the mind roll free, feelings come in. He isn't in the Richard Dawkins vein. Some of the atheists at the group he used to go to, seemed to want to take emotions out of everything. They said they didn't even want a funeral, what would be the point? When he told them about visiting the gravesite every week, they didn't understand at all. The people in the group were mostly scientists and Bob isn't particularly scientific. He doesn't consider himself a logical person, particularly. He just knows that coming here means something to him and he enjoys it.

There's always someone here, quietly doing something. Three years after Vera died, Bob spotted a chap tidying up the mound on a new grave, wanting the earth straight along the edges and nothing spilling over. Bob approached: 'Are you an engineer by any chance?' And Douglas said, 'Yes actually, a civil engineer.' Douglas had just lost his wife to cancer and Bob recommended a book of poetry that he'd found helpful after Vera died: *A Scattering*, by Christopher Reid, whose wife had also died of cancer. After they found out about the brain tumour, Bob would lie next to Vera at night trying to picture it, that repugnant thing inexorably growing in her beloved head. He could only picture something like the jellyfish he'd seen on a beach once, its large dome-shaped body with tentacles hanging down. The image of that dead jelly fish reminded Bob that the tumour had no evil schemes. It was a stupid thing, because the faster it grew, the shorter its own life would be. Soon after Vera died, Bob saw *A Scattering* reviewed and had a jolt of recognition. Reid's description of the tumour, like a squatting toad, Bob found phenomenal. *Here is somebody who knows exactly how I think*, Bob thought – *it's something squatting there, nothing evil, just something doing its job.*

Hobgoblin, nor foul fiend;
nor even the jobsworth slob
with a slow, sly scheme to rob
my darling of her mind
that I imagined;
just a tumour.

By gum, it's something when someone puts into words what you've been thinking, so you know you're not alone in what you're going through. And it's always helped Bob to remember, there was no force of evil at work in Vera's death. It is what it is.

Bob and Vera would talk about death from time to time and thought the same thing – no hell or heaven, that's it. Neither of them had been brought up with much religion. Both of their fathers had fought in World War II and after that it was – 'God? No no no.' Bob's father was in the air force and his plane came down. He broke his back and both his legs, one of which had later to be amputated. But he called that luck; the other man, his best friend, never made it out of the plane. Bob's parents didn't try to put him off religion – it was there if he wanted. He went to a Baptist Sunday school where his mum played piano, for a few years, until he got to his wild youth. There were some nice ideas at church, but they didn't sink deep.

The next time Bob saw Douglas, he passed on a copy of *A Scattering*, and Douglas became a member of their happenstance community of widowers.

Friday afternoon turned out to be quite a popular time to come, and it would be 'Hello Philip! Hello Don!' How are you doing?' 'Well, I'm not feeling so good this week.' They'd sit and chat about how they were doing with it all, and it helped. The years have dismantled this little group somewhat. The other chaps were mostly older than Bob and some have since died, though Bob still visits Philip in his care home once a fortnight. And over these ten years, he's built friendships with the groundsmen brothers, Rhys and Luke. One day, when Luke saw Bob, he came rushing over and handed him a photo. A rainbow arcing through a thunder-heavy sky. Luke had captured the moment for Bob: 'It's pointing at your wife's grave!' The fact Luke knew, of all the graves here, that the rainbow led to Vera's spot, was special. There's a gravedigger back in Vera's family tree – a Mr. Ghost. Yes, that was his real name! He was from these parts, a real tough guy, digging with a pickaxe in chalky ground, you can see how the work bulked up his shoulders. Bob tracked down a picture, framed it, and presented it to the staff, who have it on display in the cemetery's visitor room still. People come in, see the picture, 'Who's that chap?' and it starts a conversation. One of the last presents he got for Vera was a bird box for the robins in their garden. She was thrilled. So he bought one for here, too. There's the framed photograph, the bench, the bird box. He knows what he's doing – he's making a home here. And it feels nice.

He sits on her bench and thinks of the funeral celebrant's words: 'Consider the open air and the trees and look at the flowers and the grass. Listen to the sounds of the day, to the birds. They are all part of our world. Even the sound of the aircraft from Luton and the vehicles on the motorway are part of the life we know, the life of which Vera was a part. All of these things will be here when you come to visit. These places are not as frightening as many think, for they contain more love and tenderness than many parts of the world.' Vera got the day she would have wanted. They'd planned it together because she wanted quite specific things: a humanist ceremony, woodland burial, a cardboard coffin to be painted by their youngest son. The Macmillan nurse told Bob you're better off making the arrangements now, because afterwards you'll have no strength left. At the moment, you've got tons, you're rushing about because you're doing a job, you're on a roll. Once she dies, you'll go in a heap. (And that was quite right, and Bob was grateful he'd had that advice.) Bob thought to himself, *can I do this?* So, he went through the door of the undertaker's and said, 'Good morning sir, can I arrange a funeral, my wife's funeral?' 'Certainly, sir, when did she die?' 'She's not dead yet!' What an awful thing to have to do, but it was fine. He came round Monday morning for a cup of tea, Vera was sipping hers in bed. He brought along a catalogue with cardboard coffins. Their youngest son was there, too, the artist of the family, and the undertaker chap said,

'When the time comes, you can use our workshop, Scott, to paint the coffin.'

And he did. As his mum wished, he used entirely natural paints that would do no harm in the ground. Nobody but Scott and the undertakers had seen the coffin before it was carried into the hall. There was an audible intake of breath – 'Ah! How wonderful!' Most funerals, it's this horrid box that no one wants to look at. This was a different thing. A blue sky swirled with clouds on the lid and all her favourite wildflowers blooming up the sides, white, blue, red, yellow. Scott had written a little message on the top; as the coffin was being lowered in the grave, Bob saw the writing, and asked him what it said. 'I made it up, Dad.' Later, Bob had those words from the coffin carved into Vera's bench.

A couple of years before Vera got ill, Bob wasn't feeling too good himself. The doctor said he had high blood pressure and interrogated him about his lifestyle and employment. At the time, Bob was combining a job in management at a further education college with a second voluntary role and working all the hours. The doc warned if he continued that way, a few months on he'd be in trouble. He went home that night and talked over with Vera the possibility of resigning. She said that money wasn't important, recalling how she used to like the challenge of going round Sainsbury's with £5.50, adding everything up. So Bob quit, and found part time work instead, as a carer support worker, which he found both less taxing and more fulfilling than the college role. Those years were a gift, a new beginning for Bob and Vera, who had grown distant from one another during the former time of grind. Together, they redecorated their home and joined a local wildlife trust, began to learn about bats and trees and fungi. The two of them grew close again, and to top it all they welcomed their first grandchild, a girl named Leyla. Vera's diagnosis came out of the proverbial blue sky.

When they told her it was terminal lung cancer, she accepted that, and, sitting on the steps outside the hospital that day, she was very clear in what she wanted: quality over quantity of life, and to die at home – Bob could not be more grateful to the NHS team who made that Big Wish possible. Of course, it was a tough time. Her pain, her nausea, were so unbearable in those weeks after diagnosis that they looked into Dignitas. But their local GP (whom they'd known for 30 years, and who began visiting on Saturdays because he believed in 'real doctoring' that went beyond the 10-minute surgery time slot) assured them it was just a matter of finding medication that was right for Vera. Bob and Vera decided to trust him, and they got the pain under control with oxycodone – a slow-release pill twice a day with liquid top-up as required. The Macmillan nurse, too, was a wonderful human being. She answered Bob and Vera's many questions, so that they knew what to expect as the end drew nearer. 'What will happen when I die?' asked Vera. Ginette explained the practical details, the common things that happen in a dying human body, so that nothing would come as a shock to them. But she also told Vera, 'You won't die really, my dear, as long as people remember you, you'll be around still.' That really was a comfort to Vera – and to Bob and their three sons, who know now just how true those words are.

Vera wanted the family with her for her last few days, and asked Ginette to let Bob know when the time had come. In those last weeks, Bob and Vera settled into new patterns and routines, the shared ice lollies some time between 3 and 5 am, the alternating visits of day and night nurses. A memory from that time, which Bob treasures almost above all else, is how Vera would ask him to cover her, but not with her usual blue top blanket: 'I love the red blanket because it smells like you.' Vera gradually got sleepier and one day Ginette said to Bob, 'I think you'd better get the family here now.' So the three boys came, their partners, little three-month-old Leyla. Vera was happy knowing they were ok for the next generation. Something being completed, something just beginning. The family sat round Vera's bed, reading *Great Expectations* to her in relays. The book was special to her; she liked how the kind blacksmith, Joe Gargery, finds happiness with Biddy in the end.

Many people say they want to die at home, but end up in hospital because, in the final stages, the family panic. Ginette had let Bob know what to expect in Vera's last days. That she'd become unable to swallow pills and the district nurses would then provide a syringe driver. That her breathing would become jaggedy and sound awful but that it wouldn't trouble Vera. About a week before Vera died, by which time she was mostly sleeping, Bob asked Ginette whether he should move Vera's arm, which was bent over her head at what seemed an awkward angle. But Ginette said no, that was the way Vera had positioned her arm and it must not be uncomfortable to her, however it might look. Bob spent those final days lying next to Vera, drifting in and out of sleep himself, having been with her all the time for weeks and weeks by then. 'Hearing is the last sense to go,' he recalled Ginette had said, 'so talk to her, paint word pictures of calm scenes, happy times.' Towards the evening that last day, he began to hear a harshness in her breathing, and thought *ok Bob, get up, get organised*. 'I'll start talking to Mum now,' he said. He reassured her, 'Everything's fine, we're all here, Mike's here, Harry's here, Scott is here, Aisha, Leyla. Remember our narrowboat holidays on the Grand Union? How we'd relax and have a cup of tea while the boys steered and operated locks? Remember the quiet evenings? Think of the moon on the water. The water plashing gently through the reeds.' He talked about the past, interspersed with what was happening in the room. The room was getting darker, but they were there still with her, family members flowing in and out of the bedroom, flowing around her. He repeated his words, the scenes, the reassurances. Who was in the room and that everyone was alright and everything that had to be done had been done. All of the items To Be Done on Vera's clipboard had been ticked off. The night nurse came to top up Vera's pain relief; it was soon after that, she opened her eyes – which she hadn't done for several days – looked at Bob, and died.

It had all happened so quickly. On the heels of elation at the safe arrival of little Leyla in the November, Vera had mysteriously developed a feeling of incessant thirst. Just a few months later, the following March, she was gone. With the cancer diagnosis, Vera and Bob were thrown into the trenches together, only able to see as far as *right, what do we need to do next?* After she died, there was a kind of shell shock for Bob. One of the first things he set his mind to – when he became able to set his mind to anything at all – was compiling 'A Search for Meaning.'

Bob knows that any attempt at an historically accurate account is best based on primary sources. 'A Search for Meaning' is a chronological, paper-based record of Bob and Vera's final year together, built up from their diaries, emails, personal notes, and a series of daily graphs on which Bob recorded Vera's medication and jotted conversations with healthcare professionals. It is two large ring binders of 400 + pages and 180 000 words. Memory can jumble events and distort their duration. 'A Search for Meaning' helped Bob bring a sense of order to that year.

As it grew under Bob's hands, the narrative testified to Vera's interests and qualities – her unfailing courtesy to others delving into their own family histories, who would contact her seeking information and advice; her fortitude in the face of sudden serious illness and its many unpleasant symptoms. On the day of her diagnosis of incurable, inoperable lung cancer, Vera emailed a pen friend in Australia, saying she was trying to think positively – that now there'd be 'no need for false teeth or worries about old age.' That day, the young oncologist had taken them to a quiet side room and broken the news clearly, calmly. This doctor then lightened the mood by assuring Vera that the medication she was prescribing for constipation was highly effective – 'dynamite,' in fact! She spoke not as an expert from a pedestal, but as a human being. Vera delighted in this directness and repeated the dynamite joke and other gems to various friends and family members. Vera was direct herself, asking unflinching questions of her GP on his Saturday visits. When he told her, two days after her brain tumour was discovered, that her life expectancy was less than three months, she was thankful for this unambiguous information.

Putting together 'A Search for Meaning' kept Bob busy for around six months. And then what? How to live with the loneliness he found always with him, present and correct? He had to develop interests outside the house and hoped those interests could be useful. In going over the details of that last year, one of the themes to jump out was the compassionate communication and care Vera was fortunate enough to experience. The kind attentiveness of their GP, the Macmillan nurse and the hospital oncologist. The local pharmacists who took particular pride in making up prescriptions as quickly as possible. The county council social care staff who provided grab rails, a wheelchair and a special bed, promptly and without fuss. About a year after Vera died, Bob joined a local patient and public involvement group out of an impulse to give back. Since then, he's become involved with a number of other organisations. He has spoken and written many times about the many healthcare professionals who took the trouble to understand Vera's priorities and wishes and supported her to fulfil them. Bob hopes, by engaging in these ways, he may help make it possible for others to live their final chapters in the way they wish, too.

Bob prepared a copy of 'A Search for Meaning' for each of his sons. He wanted the family to appreciate the brave and open way in which Vera approached her own death. Bob's maternal grandmother died three months after he was born, and he's always found it a shame to know so little of this woman, who was a very skilful pianist and worked in the USA at a time when trans-Atlantic travel was unusual. He wanted his grandchildren – current and future – to have the chance to know their grandmother through her own words and correspondence with friends around the world.

So, 10 years now since Vera died, and Bob has just turned 70 years old, and though there may be no logical reason why these particular numbers should mean anything, they have made him stop and think. In honour of these milestones, they spent a long weekend on a narrowboat – Bob, his sons, their wives and the grandchildren, three of them by now. It was a jolly time, the boat festooned with balloons and flags. Bob shared a convivial moment with a couple of walkers on the towpath:

'Someone got a birthday?'
'Yeah, it's me!'
'We're 70 this year, too. Feels different doesn't it?'

It was the boys' idea to bring along an old album of a trip they'd taken along the same route when they were young. 'Here's a picture of Mum in front of that bridge.' So this trip they stopped in the same places and made those old photographs anew, with their kids this time. They can keep her alive, through talk of her, without tears now. Recreating those old family snaps – it is a way of holding the past and present together as one, of making peace with what time takes away and what it gives. Once the kids had gone to sleep, the grown-ups listened to some of Vera's favourite music. Radiohead, Skunk Anansie, The Eels – they've got a song Bob finds beautiful. 'It's a motherfucker/Being here without you.' When it came to the funeral, the boys said, 'You can't play that one, Dad!' It's a bit of a conundrum, isn't it? Who's the funeral for? Bob took the line it's for the people who are there, and you want music people can understand, so they went with 'Fields of Gold' and Lennon. But on her anniversaries, they listen to *her* music and remember.

Bob's new partner, Lily, doesn't get involved with occasions such as these:
    'That's your weekend for your family.'
    'But you're part of the family.'
    'No no no, I won't be there. I'm not their mum.'

When Bob and Lily were first becoming close, she asked Bob 'Can you show me your wife's grave?' So she came here, to Vera's woodland corner. Lily pointed at the bedstraw bush, with its frothy fronds that Vera loved.
    'What?'
    'Can't you see what your wife's telling you?'
The bush was heart-shaped and he'd never noticed. Since then, every Friday afternoon, Lily will press a thermos into Bob's hands and send him on his way.

10 years, 70 years. Patterns tend to mean something to us human beings. It was through family history that Vera found her place in the pattern in her last 10 years. It compelled her, this search to solve each next clue of a giant crossword puzzle that never ends. She used to find history boring as hell, but in her last year, she was teaching herself Medieval Latin to read death-bed wills. She became part of an online network of family researchers, who would exchange bits of advice and information, and find connection through some ancestor in common. The ancestors her thoughts would keep returning to were those who didn't get on well in life, who ended up in jail or transported to Tasmania just for nicking a side of bacon. The connections strung around the globe, to fellow-researchers in Australia and New Zealand, looking for pieces of their own puzzle. And the connections

threaded back into time of course, in empathetic fellowship, and there she was, a link towards the future. Vera found a sense of belonging. It made Bob proud to see her meticulous research on display at her funeral, in the printed family tree on which 7000 names stretched round the hall twice.

It's all about connection, really. Going backwards, going forwards. The bonds to those around you, whom you love, and to those further afield. There is a beauty in the interrelation of all that lives and dies. Vera's bench bears her name, but it's available, too, for other visitors to the cemetery to rest a while and contemplate. Bob's sister-in-law asked whether he would like his name added to the bench when his time comes, and he said no. He is happy to return to nature unannounced. The bench is a memorial to Vera, and its maintenance is an expression of Bob's love. Chemical varnishing is not permitted here; Bob treats the bench each year with linseed oil. After ten years, various insects have made inroads into the bench's legs. Bob will have them replaced by a craftsman friend, using offcuts from a thirty-year-old oak that grows in Bob and Vera's garden. Before he takes the bench in to the workshop, Bob wants to make it look ok, and so this afternoon he begins the task of washing, scraping, cleaning it. The bench is a memorial, yet a temporary one, and Bob knows it likely won't outlast him by too long. That's ok. As he works on it this afternoon, he finds himself reading over and pondering the words Scott thought up for his mum: 'Let me help the world to blossom a thousand times over.'

*

Many of us in the UK are choosing that, when we die, our bodies be returned to nature. Since the first woodland burial ground in the UK was established in Carlisle in 1993, more than 270 natural burial sites have sprung up around the country. Though a definition for natural burial has not yet been legally clarified, the term usually describes the burial of a body in a manner that does not inhibit decomposition, and that seeks to prevent the environmental damage that can be caused by conventional techniques. Embalming fluid, and the glues that bind chipboard coffins, often contain harmful chemicals such as formaldehyde, which is highly toxic to animals and is known to be a human carcinogen. In many cases, the aims of natural burial practitioners go beyond the prevention of environmental harm. As in the case of Sun Rising, the site Louisa chose as her husband David's final resting place, burial fees may be used to support the creation and maintenance of nature reserves, which can restore native habitat and save endangered species.

The practices of natural burial may be viewed as particularly appropriate for the non-religious, who are likely to view death as part of a natural cycle. A religious person who has been bereaved may take comfort in the idea that their loved one has now gone home to God. Those with non-religious beliefs may, like Louisa and Bob, instead find consolation in the thought that, by choosing readily biodegradable materials such as cardboard or woven willow coffins, we can give the bodies of our loved ones back to the earth, nourishing new flowers and the roots of a memorial tree that's just beginning life.

Bob and I sit together on Vera's bench in the spring sunshine. Above us, hearts of various colours and materials hang from Vera's tree. Mike and Aisha have left one on each recent visit. Bob tells me about 'A Search for Meaning.' Listening back to the recording, I can hear a hint of levity in my voice, but also a sincere desire to know, when I ask him if he's found the Meaning yet. He says his search is still ongoing. Each day, he reads the messages and diary entries from that same day of their last shared year. He re-lives those days, not in a melancholy way particularly. He tries to connect the person he is now, with who he was then.

His search is not confined to the two big ring files in his hands. There's also a digital file marked Vera on his laptop, in which he saves each letter of condolence he sends when someone he knows loses a loved one – letters that draw on what he's learnt from living through his loss of Vera. Each document is a further step in his search for meaning.

When he asks himself what it all means, sometimes he thinks of that night Vera was suddenly bolt upright at 3am, exclaiming with a beaming smile, 'Ah! The riddle is the answer!' There followed a very pleasant and relaxed discussion about why she had the answers to so many riddles but just didn't know the questions. In the end, they agreed to leave this complex topic for another day.

Bob says maybe the meaning is 'to sit here, face south, see the trees and flowers come into bloom.' I write this now with the image of Bob and Vera sitting together on the cliffs above Beer Head, sharing the quiet calm before the more chaotic years of raising their three boys. In a sense, they've circled back now, to being quietly together.

16

AN ONGOING SEARCH FOR MEANING

'We humans appear to be meaning-seeking creatures who have had the misfortune of being thrown into a world devoid of intrinsic meaning.'

Irvin Yalom, *The Gift of Therapy*

When a loved one dies, we may feel that the solid ground we used to walk upon has suddenly fallen away. We may feel that nothing in our lives makes sense or holds meaning any longer. When religious people are bereaved, some may make sense of their loss through their faith that God works all things to the good, that everything happens as it is meant to. Non-religious grievers cannot take comfort from any belief that their loss has a divinely-ordained meaning and purpose. Some of us, sometimes, may wish we could.

But Bob, who lost his wife, Vera, and Arthur, who lost his son, Ian, consider themselves fortunate to see the world as lacking God-given meaning. They know that religious beliefs can be more harmful than helpful. Religious grievers may struggle with feelings of anger towards God, believe they are being punished, wonder why their prayers went unanswered, or worry that their loved ones may be in hell. The questions 'Why me? Why us?' can add to the burden of loss. When someone with a religious belief loses a loved one, especially when the loss is sudden, violent or untimely, that person's assumptions about the world may be shattered; they may have previously had faith that events are orchestrated by a benevolent and just creator and may struggle to reconcile their experiences with these prior assumptions. They may have previously felt protected by a belief that 'God doesn't give you more than you can handle,' but then have to handle more than it feels possible to bear. One recent study compared outcomes amongst bereaved religious believers and atheists and found that the religious grievers overall had higher levels of psychological distress and complicated grief. Complicated grief is a term sometimes used to describe grief that continues to be unusually intense, and to dominate the bereaved person's life, more than six months on from a loss.

When Arthur and Bob shared their stories with me, I was powerfully struck by the lightness they found in their naturalistic view of the world. They were free from 'Why me? Why us?' They were not weighed down by wondering if they were suffering because they deserved to suffer, because some higher force had decided they should suffer. Arthur was grateful to have no anger regarding his son's death at the age of 29. He did not need to rage at God for cutting Ian's life short; he was able to accept that it was simply bad luck. Bob understood that Vera's tumour was not vindictive; it simply did what tumours do. There is a randomness to the processes of life and of disease. There is a kind of sense to be made, simply through the understanding that we cannot expect life and death always to make any larger kind of sense.

Some non-religious people do view the world as imbued with intrinsic meaning; they may not believe in God or gods, but may still believe in some form of higher life force and that 'everything happens for a reason.' However, research shows that non-religious people are more likely than those with religious beliefs to agree with the statement, 'Life is only meaningful if you provide the meaning yourself.' When Vera and Ian died, Bob and Arthur rebuilt their lives with self-made meanings.

We make choices about how to tell the story of what we've lived through. Arthur holds onto the assurance that Ian had many good and even great days even during the year they lived with cancer. He finds meaning in the fact that money raised in Ian's name has helped many families to share good and great days together away from Cancerland. Arthur and Wendy's life now is not the one they hoped for, but they choose to find continuing value in the present and future they can still share, the new memories they can make on the open road. When Bob looked back through 'A Search for Meaning,' his record of all that happened in his and Vera's last shared year, he found a number of meanings in its pages. He found a portrait of Vera's generosity and courage, to show their sons and grandchildren; he found the kindness and compassion of the many people who supported them through Vera's final chapters; and he found a new personal impetus to pay that generosity and kindness forwards.

I am one of those people who believes life is only meaningful if you provide the meaning yourself. Sometimes I struggle to provide that meaning. No one ever asked me to write this book and at times it has been difficult to hold onto a belief it's worth continuing. But when I am searching for meaning, I instinctively turn to stories – to reading, hearing and telling them. It is wonderful when those who share their stories with me, let me know that doing so, and reading my account of their experiences, has been meaningful for them. Linda, whom we met in chapter 5 said that talking through with me her experiences of loss and illness helped her make some useful connections for herself. Bob thanked me for taking care to capture his thoughts and feelings precisely. Arthur was pleased I'd put so much of his son, Ian, in my piece. If my book has reached your hands, I hope it means something to you, too.

17

ROGER

and the treasure chest of memories

Roger had several years to get used to the idea of being without his mum. He began to lose her long before she died. He and his brother look quite alike so when he visited his mum, she'd ask him about his brother's wife, of whom she was particularly fond: 'Where's Bethan today?' To begin with he'd say 'I'm Roger – I'm not Pete, I'm Roger.' But with Alzheimer's, the advice is just to go along with what they say, don't contradict, don't challenge, just be with someone and go along. So then, when his mum asked about Bethan, Roger would reply 'Oh, she's at home baking,' or 'Look at the lovely weather! She's gardening today,' and his mum would say 'That's nice, dear!' Then one day she called him Roger and he thought, *my goodness, there's something of her left.*

When one of his best friends died from AIDS, it was his first bereavement and it was terrible and Roger thought *I never want to go through that again.* He wanted to love people and be close, but he never wanted to repeat that awful shock of loss. One thing he learned that helped was the idea of a treasure chest of memories. It helps, when someone's died, to have precious shared experiences to look back on. Roger tried to make things nice for his mum – he took her for walks, car rides, they'd have little jokes about things. Sometimes the two of them would sit together on a bench that overlooked a lovely pond, taking in the ripples and the lily pads, the shimmering blue dragonflies. Roger wanted to keep his mum's quality of life as good as possible. But he was also consciously creating special experiences and storing them away for himself, so that later, when he opened up that chest, all those moments would be sparkling up at him.

When a loved one dies, they are no longer with us physically; like Roger, all who lose a loved one must face a future without that person at their side. We may sometimes envy those who believe that in a life to come they'll hold their loved ones in their arms again. Those of us who can't believe in that kind of eternal life may, in time, though, begin to take some comfort from the 'symbolic immortality' of our loved one, who continues to live in us and in the world.

Humanist author Arthur Dobrin has written that one of the 'ultimate comforts for the bereaved' is 'the recognition that the great mystery is not death but birth, not that someone loved is now gone but that the person was here at all.' Ann Druyan expressed a similar sentiment following the death of her husband, physicist Carl Sagan. She noted that because of his famously atheistic views, people often approached her to ask whether at the end, Carl converted to a belief in the afterlife, and whether she thought she would see him again. She told them that her husband 'faced his death with unflagging courage and never sought refuge in illusions.' She said, 'I don't think I'll ever see Carl again. But I saw him. We saw each other. We found each other in the cosmos, and that was wonderful.'

Death may erase a shared future we have hoped for and imagined, but the fact of love remains. As Louisa observed, following the death of her beloved David, the fact of a shared happiness still stands. Many of those who shared their stories for this book told me of the comfort they take from treasured memories of their lost loved one. Arthur has those match days with his best football buddy, Ian. Bob has the family holidays on the canal, the quiet evenings he spent with his wife Vera, looking at the moon on the water as the boys slept. Others may be able to bring us treasures, too. Once a loved one has gone, there are no new memories to be made with them, but perhaps someone approaches us in the street and shares a memory, or writes in a condolence card something that we never knew. So now we have a new piece of our loved one to hold onto.

The feeling that our loved ones live on in us and in the world in some way can be consoling, particularly when the person who has died has lived a long, full life. Even though Arthur's son, Ian, died just short of his 29th birthday, Arthur and Wendy have still been able to find some comfort in memories of their shared years and in knowing their son was much-loved by his friends. But I began to wonder, what comfort can there be when a life is even shorter? How do non-religious people cope with losing someone who is very young?

18

AN ENDING WHEN WE'D JUST BEGUN

my story, iii

The sonographer frowns. She isn't seeing what she was expecting – the outline of a foetus at 12 weeks' gestation. My eyes flick between the screen and her face as she searches deeper. Then it appears. A little jellybean shape.

'I'm sorry to tell you there's no heartbeat. This embryo stopped developing at around 6 weeks.'

We go into another room, waiting for someone to speak to us about what happens next. A student nurse comes in, with a wide smile, not knowing what has happened. Niko takes my hand. My body hasn't known to let this pregnancy go, so I'm going to need a procedure – a D&C – to 'evacuate the products of conception.' We'd been expecting to go home with the first images of our baby to show my family, whom I've already told the happy news. We leave with nothing and I send today's news by text because I don't feel like talking. Niko and I hold each other on the sofa.

Four months earlier, another shared experience had unfolded here. We were lying together one evening. Niko could feel my heart beating hard and fast and was worried something was very wrong. I was only nervous because I'd decided to ask him to marry me. Niko had a failed marriage behind him; I knew marrying again wasn't a priority for him. But eight months after meeting, we'd moved in together and he'd asked if maybe we should have a baby. I wanted that very much, but liked the idea of being married first, so without his knowing, I bought him a ring, gold, cut intricately through with a tree stretching its branches up and out.

He said 'Of course,' and though the ring wasn't a good fit for his ring finger, it didn't matter. He slid it on his other hand.

We planned for a seaside wedding in April. It didn't take much planning because we wanted something small and simple. Then when we went away for our first Christmas together, I forgot to take my birth control pills with me. We didn't conceive that month, but we thought *why bother going on the pill again?* In January, we conceived. At my first appointment with the midwife, I was given an October due date. I had my wedding dress made with a little leeway for a thirteen-week bump. We flew to Bulgaria so I could meet Niko's parents for the first time; I'd learnt the Bulgarian for 'I'm pregnant, 10 weeks.' We celebrated with an Easter lunch of eggs with shells dyed red. There's a traditional game a bit like conkers but with eggs – the one whose egg remains uncracked will have robust health for the coming year. I won that game. I told my family early on about the baby, too, in part to explain why I wasn't going to have a hen do or drink champagne on my wedding day. I felt an element of disbelief that I had a baby growing inside me. It had all happened so fast. We'd only known each other a year. But we were happy.

And now, the week before our wedding we're told there isn't going to be a baby in October after all. I feel stupid, as though I've fallen for a trick. I've been telling people I'm pregnant, thinking of myself as pregnant, and now I'm not. I'm told they can book the D&C in for the following morning, but I choose to schedule it for three days' time, because I don't teach on Fridays. I don't want to inconvenience my colleagues or have what I'm going through be public knowledge. It feels strange to go to work the next day as normal, knowing I'm carrying something small and dead inside me.

Niko takes me into hospital on the Friday morning. I know there will be a wait of several hours and tell him not to stay. I quite like the idea of a few hours reading by myself. My book is Julian Barnes' *The Sense of an Ending*. When they wheel me in for the op, the nurse distracts me with questions about my life, while slapping the back of my hand with slight brutality to bring up a blood vessel for the cannula. The last thing I hear is 'The tide is high but I'm holding on'…Then I open my eyes again and ask whether or not it's over, because I have a disorienting feeling no time has passed at all.

It is over. Niko takes me home. When, recently, I went back through old emails to check my memory of the timeline, I found a confirmation of my Pizza Hut delivery order. Pizza! Of course pizza is what got me through that day.

My family ask whether we still want to go ahead with the wedding the following week. We never have any doubt we do. I contact the manager of the restaurant where we're having our reception to tell her I'll be able, after all, to eat and drink whatever I like on the day. The weather forecast is laughable – it will be a dry and sunny week with the exception of that one day. The forecast is accurate - gales tear at the pier where we have our post-lunch walk. Rain drums on the roof where we have our reception dinner. It doesn't matter. We drink champagne. I am still bleeding on our wedding night, but I have married the man I love with my family around me.

The hospital tells me they think I've had a 'complete molar pregnancy,' but they're going to send the 'products of conception' off for analysis by the experts at Charing Cross. My online searches later leave me confused about how to think of what has happened to me. I read that if you have a 'complete mole,' no parts of a baby form. Only 'molar tissue' develops in the womb. This happens when a sperm from the father fertilises an empty egg. Was this only ever a mutant ball of cells and never a potential person? And why do I have empty eggs?

I am also told that in some cases, a molar pregnancy leads to a kind of cancer developing. I will need to be monitored by the Charing Cross Gestational Trophoblast Disease Service. It is an adjustment: I'm not having a baby. I might have cancer. Every two weeks, they send me test kits in the post, which I have to take to my GP surgery. The receptionist sees the word 'oncology' on the box and looks at me gravely. They have to check my blood and urine to see whether my hormone levels are falling back to normal. If my HCG levels remain high, that could indicate a tumour, requiring chemotherapy.

At a follow-up hospital appointment they tell me actually I've had a partial molar pregnancy, not a complete. With a partial molar pregnancy, there is an excess of genetic material: three sets of chromosomes. It happens when two sperm fertilise an egg at the same time. An embryo can begin to develop, but along with it an abnormal cell mass grows, which rapidly overcomes the developing baby. With this news, my situation shifts again. What I saw on the sonographer's screen – that jellybean with its curving line round from a hint of a head to a hint of a body – had been the beginnings of a person after all. That outline was the visible intention of a baby. Our intention.

Like many who have experienced a loss, I try to make sense of it, I look for answers. Online, I find out that being on oral contraceptives soon before conceiving increases the risk of a molar pregnancy. The exact reason why this should be the case is unknown. When I stopped taking the pill, I'd been aware of advice to wait three months before trying to conceive. I'd checked why and was told it can take a few cycles for periods to fall back into a regular pattern, so waiting a few months to conceive makes it easier to accurately determine a conception date. I knew that scans are pretty accurate in determining a foetus' gestation anyway. We didn't want to wait to start our family. Of course, if anyone had ever told us that the pill has been linked to increased risk of an unsurvivable genetic abnormality, we would have done things differently.

*

When I set out to write this book, I didn't intend to write about my miscarriage. We didn't name this baby, never met this baby. It hardly even feels legitimate to think or speak of a baby in this pregnancy. The genetic abnormality meant the cells that started on the process of division and multiplication could never have become a person. I have been quite dismissive with myself about this loss.

But if a friend told me she'd had a miscarriage, would I be dismissive? Would I be thinking *that's nothing that matters*. Of course I wouldn't. A friend did tell me about her miscarriage, when the experience was still very recent and raw. I hugged her and we both had tears in our eyes. So yes, it hurt, it mattered, that Niko and I wanted a child, but the child could not be.

19

CLAIRE

and secular support when a baby dies

When we lose a close one, many of us are fortunate enough to be able to lean on the support of a loving group of family and friends. In some situations, we may also feel the need of the more specialised support offered by bereavement services.

In the UK, around 15 babies die before, during, or soon after birth every day. For parents who have lost a baby, the availability of sensitive and appropriate support is critical. Many hospitals offer baby funerals for late miscarriages, stillbirths and in cases when a baby has died shortly after birth. David Savage, in his recent guide to non-religious pastoral care, observes that 'hospital funeral ceremonies for babies are usually conducted by a hospital chaplain.' These chaplains 'are likely to be ordained members of a Christian church, yet most mothers will be non-religious,' as 56% of people aged 34-44 are non-religious and 61% of people aged 25-34. Since the latest information shows that 68% of 18-24-year-olds belong to no religion, the need for secular support in hospitals and other settings is only going to become more pressing in future. Savage urges that hospitals 'should ensure that people with non-religious beliefs are offered a funeral conducted by a humanist or non-religious celebrant on the same basis that they offer funerals to people with Christian beliefs conducted by Christian clergy. Funerals conducted by religious hospital chaplains should not be the default position for non-religious baby funerals.'

Some hospitals offer secular support to bereaved families, separately from chaplaincy, in the form of specialist bereavement counselling or therapy. An audit conducted jointly by the charities Sands (the Stillbirth and Neonatal Death Charity) and Bliss, published in 2018, found that 83% of neonatal units have access to at least one staff member whose role includes offering support to bereaved parents. However, worryingly, in only 14% of cases does that staff member have dedicated time in their workplan to provide that support. Claire, who worked as a counsellor with bereaved parents at an East London Hospital between 1999 and 2014, told me what a difference it can make to bereaved parents to receive support that is in keeping with their worldview.

Claire's role came out of a piece of research looking at long term psychological outcomes following miscarriage, with patients who'd had someone come and sit down on the bed and let them talk, and those who hadn't had that. It was found that when a nurse had taken the trouble to sit and tell the patient 'It's ok to talk about how you're feeling,' those were the patients who did better long term. So the hospital decided to set up a counselling service. Claire had worked for many years as a nurse and then trained as a therapist, making the role a good fit for her. She worked with patients who'd had miscarriages or stillbirths, or whose babies had died soon after birth.

She would work within the client's frame of reference, so sometimes a bereaved mother might say 'My grandmother died last year and I believe she's looking after my baby,' and Claire might say 'And does that give you comfort?' The mum would say it did, and talk about how and why. Claire might then say 'So I'm guessing you also believe at some stage you'll be joining them?' And the mum would say 'Yes, that makes it easier to bear.' For Claire, that was fine, if that worldview was a resource a patient could draw upon at a difficult time. When a baby died, Claire would always send a midwife to ask whether the parents would like to see her. Sometimes when counselling was offered, parents would decline and say 'I'll go to see the vicar,' or 'I'll speak to the imam' instead. Often, it was parents with non-religious beliefs who chose to see Claire. Usually, what the parents wanted most was for another person to acknowledge that their child existed. As soon as a pregnancy begins, if it's a wanted pregnancy, you begin to imagine yourself months hence, pushing the pram, holding your child. Both parents live with that child through pregnancy, and it's all very real as the baby grows and they speak to her, or play music to him. Parents grieve a future they'll no longer have. Claire could be with them through that, and if the couple had another pregnancy, Claire would offer counselling through that time too; she'd hear their fears and all the muddled feelings that the prospect of another child could bring up.

An additional part of Claire's role was to train midwives on working with parents after a baby dies. She talked about everything from the moment you discover there's no heartbeat – what you say and do, what's appropriate and what's not. Many of the midwives were deeply religious and didn't realise the negative impact that their comments sometimes had on parents who didn't share their views. Claire printed out a list of things that patients had told her had been said to them. Things like 'She's with God now,' or 'God will give you another child.' Even when such words are intended to be supportive, if they don't fit with the parents' beliefs, hearing these things can add to the loss, to the sense of being lost. Claire would always tell the midwives, 'You may talk to God about your patients, but don't talk to patients about God.' She had to take on one of the hospital chaplains who was visiting bereaved patients without their asking him. He'd bowl in and take his God in with him, and Claire had a number of patients who told her they'd found this very intrusive and upsetting. In the last years that Claire was in post, the training sessions ground to a halt because management wouldn't allow staff the necessary time away from the ward. Claire noticed some of those unfortunate behaviours start to creep back, as a new generation of nurses came in whom she hadn't trained.

Claire hopes though, looking back, that the work she did was something worthwhile. There were people who told her 'I never thought I'd get through this, I couldn't have done it without you.' You think *of course you could,* but also, you give yourself a pat and think *good job, well done.* When they come back and they've had another baby and the baby's thriving, it's all very wonderful. When it's all gone well, and they're not depressed and you saw them through that, it's a special feeling.

After speaking to Arthur and to Claire, I still wanted to understand more about what it is like to lose a much-loved child and how non-religious parents can manage to move forward from such a great loss. Part of me recoiled from thinking about child loss, surely one of the hardest things to go through. Another part of me felt that if I wanted this book to be of use to anyone, I needed to be willing to look deeply and directly at the hardest possibilities. Through Child Bereavement UK, I reached out to non-religious parents bereaved of a baby or child. Kim offered to tell me about her daughter, May.

20

KIM

when we look at the stars, we'll think of her

Kim's first pregnancy had gone smoothly and resulted in a healthy little girl called Lizzie. Two years later, second time round, the medics sort of left Kim to it and didn't really keep a close eye on how the pregnancy was going. The first sign of anything wrong came on the day she thought she might be going into labour. She went into hospital and got sent for a scan. Kim was huge, but it turned out this was mostly due to excess fluid. The baby in her womb was much smaller than expected. As soon as Kim gave birth, baby May was whisked away to be intubated as she couldn't swallow or breathe unaided. She went for surgery at another hospital at just one day old. Tests were done to determine what was wrong, and it took five long days for a diagnosis to be confirmed. May had Edwards' syndrome – a condition described as 'incompatible with life,' which is not a great thing for a mum and dad to hear.

She did have a life, though it was a short one. She opened her eyes. Kim knew when May was upset, when she was hungry, and when she was a bit more settled. All day, every day, Kim sat holding May's hand or foot or whatever of her was exposed at the time, and they were connected. With the diagnosis came the news there was nothing to be done except remove her tubes and see if she could survive without them. It was highly unlikely she'd be able to. The next morning, on the eighth day of May's life, Kim remembers her husband saying 'Right, come on, let's do this, let's do May proud.' And it was really important that the two of them were shoulder to shoulder. May's tubes were taken out, and she was brought to Kim and Dan. Kim held her in her arms for an hour and a half. When it became clear that she had taken her last breaths, Dan went to get the doctor, to record May's time of death. The staff wanted to put her in a pretty dress or whatever, and Kim said 'You can do that, but don't do it here.' She and Dan both felt the same: this wasn't any longer May, just what was left.

Kim was brought up broadly C of E in the same way that lots of people are, in that they don't really know what they believe. As a teenager, she was a bit of a goth, took an interest in the paranormal and 'Are ghosts real?' But as she gained a scientific education, it became 'Well, I'll believe anything if I can see it,' and she never did see anything that made the Christian story plausible to her, nor any reason to be told what to do by an organisation with a lot of money and power – especially male power. Dan had a similar upbringing and had formed similar atheistic views. Now, they had to take advice very quickly on how to explain May's death to two-year-old Lizzie. Children can be very traumatised if Mum and Dad come home from hospital without the person that was there. They didn't want to tell her any lies, but they wanted to say something that would help her understand and provide some comfort. Kim told Lizzie 'May died, which means she's gone away, but when we look at the stars, that's when we'll think of her.' So, to Lizzie, May has always been a star. After Kim went back to work, her mother-in-law took care of Lizzie. On the drive home at the end of the day, Lizzie would be looking up and asking 'Which star is May? Where do you think May is?' That was nice for Lizzie to think about.

But Kim didn't see May up in the stars. The gap, the absence, all the stuff that wasn't going to happen, hit her very early. Your child's imagined future is conjured up in pregnancy – where they'll go to school, what will be their favourite things to do. When your baby dies, you lose more than just your baby: you lose the child, teenager and adult they were going to be. This was 19 years ago – it is 19 years since May died. It was not like in the 50s or 60s when, if a baby died, the world pretended that child did not exist. Hospitals were starting to understand the importance of making memories when a child's life is likely to be very short, so that parents will have *something* to take home, when they can't take home their child. These were the days before digital photography, so the hospital staff took Polaroids of May, in case the pictures on Kim's camera film didn't work out. When May was intubated, she had plasters holding the tubes in place. There was a lovely nurse one day, taking a plaster off, who turned to Kim and said 'Normally I'd throw this away. Do you want me to throw this away?' and Kim said, 'No no, I really want it.' Kim and Dan put together a memory box, in which they kept this plaster, some of May's hair, what she was wearing when she died, a teddy: everything and anything that came near her during her life, even the eye mask she wore when she had to be under bright lights. When May was diagnosed, Kim and Dan were given a printout of the results from her DNA test – it was a visual confirmation she had 47 instead of the usual 46 chromosomes, the extra 18th chromosome confirming Edwards' syndrome. They had it framed and hung it on the wall at home. For some reason, it felt even more special to Kim and Dan than May's hand and footprints did. Being shown the image of May's chromosomes destroyed their world at the time, but it is *her*, it's like her signature.

Though Kim had been clear that May's dead body wasn't *her*, for some reason it was important to have something to spread or bury. She was warned that when a baby is cremated there may be no remains, no ashes to take away. So they chose burial for May. Kim's dad offered to organise drinks for the funeral and Kim asked him to get champagne. At first he said 'That isn't how we do things,' but Kim said 'Can you please just treat it like it's her 18th? I want it to feel like that because we're never going to get that.' On the day of the funeral, people weren't sure about intruding on their grief, but Kim's dear friend Iris, appointed as her mouthpiece for the day, said 'Please come back to the house, you're all welcome.' Kim wanted to hear people chatting, glasses clinking. She wanted a full house – a fullness instead of an absence. And because Kim had such lovely friends, and they wanted to do what they could to help, they went along with it.

Kim used to work near the hospital where May was born. For a few years after May died, she would go in her lunch break, to help train the staff in how to deal with people who are losing a baby. It was one of the ways in which she coped with May not being with her: she thought, *even if you aren't here, your presence will be felt in this hospital.* Medical staff are there to make us better, but they don't always do it! May was born on an ordinary maternity ward, where staff are mostly used to life, and they didn't know what to say or how to deal with Kim. After Kim gave birth, May was taken away very quickly, and Dan went with her. The midwife said to Kim, 'Just wait here a second, I need to pop out.' Kim was left alone, not knowing where her baby was, or whether she was still alive. She found out later the midwife had been struggling with her own feelings and had gone to make herself a cup of tea! After Kim raised what had happened, the hospital changed their policy so that a woman who's just given birth should never be left alone. If a midwife needs a break, they must first call someone else to be there. At Kim's six-week post-natal check, the doctor said 'You're young, you can have another – just take a holiday, relax and have a go,' and it was at that point Kim walked out. No one would tell a recent widow 'You're still young and attractive – you can marry again.' When Kim went to help train the hospital staff, she'd say back to them the things that had been said to her. It would be 'Here's what not to say, here's what you might consider doing.' She told them how she'd felt completely lost and all she wanted was for someone to put a hand on her arm and say 'I'm really sorry about what's happening.'

People didn't know what to say to her. If the person who has died has lived a full life, there are good times to reminisce about. What is there to say about a child who never even made it home from hospital? When you see someone in the street they can't say 'I'll always remember that time when she…' So maybe that someone will cross to the other side instead. Soon after May died, a friend of Kim's was hosting a Body Shop party at her house and Dan said, 'Go, it will be nice for you and I'll look after Lizzie.' A lady was there with a baby, maybe two or three months old. She held the child out to Kim saying, 'Do you mind just holding him a minute?' and went off to the kitchen. It was lovely for Kim to hold a baby and she was proud of how she was keeping herself together; he was a boy and didn't look like May at all, so it felt ok. Kim saw her friend talking to the baby's mum, perhaps saying something like 'It's lovely to see Kim holding a baby – this is what has happened.' The mum strode back, took him off Kim and said, 'He's my baby, you can't have him, you've got death on you.' Kim left soon after. (Years later, when *Eastenders* ran a plot where Ronnie takes Kat's baby, Kim wrote in saying 'People think women who've lost a baby want someone else's baby. We don't – we want our own baby!')

But Kim did find people who understood. There was an online group for parents of children with Edwards' syndrome. It was mostly people in the USA, and they were very direct, very gushing in their support. Because it was the early days still of the internet, it wasn't overwhelming, there weren't thousands of posts a day – you'd go online and find the same person and say, 'This thing happened today,' and it helped to feel you weren't alone. Kim didn't see herself as a support group person at all, but she persuaded herself to go along to a Sands meeting, about four months after May died. People were arriving and just chatting: 'Oh, I can't believe I got a parking fine' and things like that. It was the weirdest thing – Kim was thinking *I know you're all here because you've had a baby die. Why are you being normal?* Something clicked in Kim: *Oh! I will get normal again then.* Sands was great – how wonderful to talk about what happened with May and have a stranger say, 'Could you tell me a bit more? I'd really like to hear about your daughter.' It felt good to hear other parents' stories too, although those stories were very sad. Before losing May, Kim had tended to close herself off from anyone she felt was not her kind of person. But losing May, and meeting others who'd also been through something very hard, opened her up to the possibilities in people. She began to listen to people more carefully, and to feel more compassion.

Through Sands, Kim met another bereaved mother, Samantha, who also wanted to help improve the local hospital for families of the future. They heard that the hospital had been allocated some money specifically to improve maternity services, so Kim contacted the head of midwifery to discuss its use. Most of it had to go on a new roof, but what was left – along with additional funds that Kim and Samantha raised – went towards two new side rooms. When you don't have your baby, you don't want to be on a ward with mothers who do. Kim and Samantha worked with the hospital to design two rooms for women whose babies are unwell or have died, so they could have somewhere quiet. Samantha named one room the Rainbow Room in memory of her daughter who had died; Kim chose the Star Room as May's legacy. It was so lovely, recently, watching a TV programme filmed at the hospital, to spot that a midwife assistant was walking out of May's room.

A year and a bit after May died, Kim had Esther. Lizzie and Esther have grown up knowing that because of their sister, May, other people's lives are better. There are women who have had more compassionate doctors because of May; parents whose experiences in hospital have been a little more calm and kind. Kim and Dan both agreed that May should be a presence in their home, and in their lives. They've always had pictures of May up in the house – including one of Lizzie meeting her little sister – and they've spoken openly about her. They have stars in their home – on a tea light here, a bowl there. One piece of advice that Kim was given early on was 'Don't have fixed rituals, because if you break them, you'll feel terrible.' So they never said 'We'll go to her grave every Sunday,' or whatever. Kim didn't want her surviving children to feel guilt, to feel like they didn't care as much about their sister as they should. But, on Christmas Eve, Lizzie and Esther never wanted to be anywhere other than their own beds, so including May that day each year was workable. They're usually in their pyjamas for most of Christmas Eve, but they'll always take a walk to May's grave and put a little Christmas tree there. When the girls were younger, they used to put a marble or something small they thought May might like, and it was a nice way to keep her memory alive for them. It was very important to Lizzie that they should have a birthday party for May, and that there should be cake – it might have been mainly the cake that was important! These days, they usually go out for a family dinner for May's birthday, just as they would for Lizzie and Esther.

Five years ago, Kim's dear friend Iris died. After May died, Iris was great. She was straight round to the house: 'Right, I'll take Lizzie out,' and 'I can do this and that.' May's death brought them even closer than they had been. These days Kim goes to tend both May's and Iris' graves, not often, but from time to time. And when she goes, she talks to them – not because she thinks they can hear her, but just because somehow it would seem rude to visit and say nothing. She'll say things like, 'Oh, you're looking messy, let's clean you up.' When Kim's had problems that Iris would have understood, she's said 'It's really inconvenient that you're not here;' she'll go to the grave and say something like that, and she wouldn't talk to Iris anywhere else but there, which is ridiculous when she thinks about it, and she can't really explain it, but that's how it is.

Iris died around Christmas time, totally without warning. An aneurism burst inside her brain. Kim had been expecting to see Iris the next day for Christmas drinks. She felt some urge to go and see her body, but Iris's husband said 'Are you really sure you want to do that?' and Kim said 'Actually no, I really don't, it won't be Iris any more.' When you're gone, you're gone. Kim's youngest daughter Esther gets a bit spooked by Halloween, and Kim said to her 'Look, May's died, my mother-in-law died soon after, my dad's died, and my best friend who was like my sister – *none* of them have made any attempt, there's never been anything from any of them, so I just don't believe it.' Kim is certain that Iris would have come back if she could. She'd have had plenty to say! But she didn't come and she didn't speak. It was a final separation.

Kim had the same panicked realisation soon after the deaths of both May and Iris: 'I can't remember what her face looks like!' There's a song she loves but still can't listen to now because it has the line 'I'm worried I'll forget your face.' Kim arranged Iris's funeral along with Hazel, a friend Iris knew from church. Kim said to Hazel, 'I envy you having your faith to fall back on, having that belief you'll see the ones you love again.' But Hazel said 'I'm not coping well *because* of my faith. Why would God take her? She's got three children, she was just a brilliant person, and I'm really struggling with it. I'm having a lot of conversations with God at the moment.' Iris herself had been religious – she believed in prayers and heaven. Six weeks before she died, she lost her grandfather and said 'Well, at least he's in heaven now with Grandma.' Kim thought *that's nice, isn't it, to think like that.* She can see how those kinds of thoughts could comfort. But when it doesn't quite fit it must be hard in your head to square that circle. At Iris's funeral, the focus of the vicar's sermon was 'She's gone home, she's now at home with God.' Lizzie and Esther, 16 and 13 at the time, were just furious afterwards, saying 'She's got a home with her children, why does God want her with him?' And yeah, it did seem like this guy was having to work hard to explain why someone, at 42 – who dedicated herself to other people, who had three young kids who needed her – why his God had seen fit to take her.

Iris always had immaculate nails. After she died, Kim went out and bought some very nice nail varnish – the base coat and the top coat and all the stuff you need – and on a Sunday night she'd do her nails. After about two years, she went to see someone to say 'What's wrong with my nails?' because they kept splitting, and the lady said 'Your nails can't cope with varnish, you've got to stop.' So that little ritual came to an end. Grieving for Iris was different from grieving for May. With May, Kim misses what she never had, whereas with Iris, she misses what she did have. She can still hear Iris' laugh and smell her perfume. She doesn't have that with May. The analogy Kim would use for her bereavement journeys – both with Iris and May – is that it's like the formation of a scar. For the first however-long, the wound is bleeding, painful, open to infection by people being thoughtless, or anything happening that isn't what you want to happen that day. Over time, a bit of skin grows over – though it still hurts if you touch it. Later, it's there and if you know about it, you can see it's there, but you think of it less often. Kim used to get May's memory box out every birthday, but she doesn't any more; she doesn't really feel the need, though the fact it's there is still important. Up till Lizzie was eight or nine, they'd go on walks and drop in at the graveyard to say hello to May on the way home. Now it's usually just at Christmas and her birthday. If someone had asked Kim 17 years ago how many children she has, she'd have said 'I've had three. I've got two.' You realise quite quickly that's not the kind of answer most people are ready to hear. Now, if someone asks, she'll probably just say 'Two.' She'll talk about May, though, if something comes up. She's old enough to have stopped fearing other people's embarrassment. People do get embarrassed and that's alright, you can put them at ease and say 'It's ok, it's just part of my history.' Lizzie and Esther feel ok talking about May, too. When their friends come round and see pictures of May and don't quite know what to say, the girls lead by example and say 'This is May, this is my sister who died.' Then it's out there and it's normal. For the girls, May's still a member of the family. Esther is applying to study design at university. As part of her portfolio, she's used May's 'signature' for a jewellery design: the bands of May's 18th chromosomes are replicated in beads, to form a bracelet.

Recently a friend called Kim to say her sister-in-law had just had a stillborn baby: 'I don't know what to do with Amy, what do I do, what do I not do?' Kim said, 'Give her my number, if she'd like to speak to me she can.' When she put the phone down, Kim thought *ooh, I don't know if I should be doing this* – because you can be trained as a Sands befriender, but Kim hadn't had that training. Actually, it was fine when Amy called – it was an upsetting conversation for Kim, but nice to feel that she could help. Just to be able to say to Amy, 'What you're saying now is what I was saying, and you think you're going mad but you're not and don't think about tomorrow, just get on with today and tomorrow will come later.' It was nice for Kim to feel she could reassure someone; it was also interesting to remember quite how bad she'd been back then, how she used to think and feel in the early days after losing May, and how she's been able to put her grief into a place where it's more manageable. When a baby dies, there aren't many people to share your grief with, not many people knew and loved the person that you lost, and perhaps that's partly why the healing goes much slower. It's manageable now, but it never goes, it really never goes.

The day before May's birthday is always hard, because Kim's got nothing that she needs to do, no presents needing to be wrapped or banners to put up. For Lizzie and Esther, Kim's always taken care to make the day special, so they feel like a Birthday Queen, but there isn't anything she can do for May. Even this year, 19 years on, Kim went to bed crying the night before May's birthday, because in the day-to-day she's used to May not being here, but the thought that May should be turning a year older is hard to bear. It takes a long time to get over the life that isn't there, and perhaps you never do. The gap between Lizzie and Esther, where May should be, still feels like a physical thing.

The world looked different to Kim after May died. She saw how insignificant we are, and that time respects no one. May lived for an hour and a half after coming out of the incubator; Kim wanted that time to go on forever, and it didn't. As she and Dan drove out of the hospital with their lives broken, to go and tell their daughter that her sister had just died, nobody cared, nobody knew. It wasn't etched on their faces like they thought it was. The road was very busy; Dan was struggling to pull out and they got beeped, he was going 'Just let us!...' and Kim was thinking *we can't get a break.* It took two hours to do a journey that should have taken 30 minutes and she was thinking *yeah, we're not as important as we thought we were, and there's definitely no one looking out for us.* But it was actually quite freeing to realise that you just have to get on with doing what you're doing and the world will carry on around you.

And it is a beautiful world. After May died, Kim began to notice things she hadn't really seen before. The leaves turning colour, a sunset, a rainbow, a starry night – all looked completely different to her and they still do now.

About ten years ago, Kim heard physicist Carl Sagan explain how the elements that form our DNA, our teeth, our blood, came into being within collapsing stars: we're starstuff. It's poetry and science at the same time. It hadn't been too fanciful, then, to tell two-year-old Lizzie all those years back, 'When we look at the stars, we'll think of May.'

21

11:11 AND OTHER MOMENTS IN TIME

my story, iv

Two months after getting married, at the end of my summer term of teaching, Niko and I go away together. The remote Scottish island has only two permanent residents, and their house is on the opposite side from our little honeymoon cottage. We overlook a bay where seals bob up and the water is bracing still in late June.

This is a place to be together away from everything else, but I can't totally get away. I'm waiting for my test results. So far, since miscarrying a partial molar pregnancy, my levels of the pregnancy hormone HCG have been going downwards, but not as quickly as anyone would like. The risk of a cancerous tumour developing still looms.

There's no mobile reception in our cottage. I have to climb to the island's highest point to make the call for my latest results. It's good news – my HCG level is now nearly back in normal range. If this continues, within a few months we could be cleared to try for another baby.

But I notice something else while on the island. At the centre of vision in my right eye, there's a cloudy patch. I am 32 years old. A visit to the optician and a referral to Moorfield's later, I find out I need surgery to remove a cataract, a procedure more usually performed on people in their seventies and eighties. Everyone is puzzled. As a risk-averse person who's never broken a bone, I've managed to stay out of hospital, and now, within a year, I need two operations.

There's a waiting time, though, of several months. My operation is scheduled for the following spring. Since it's inadvisable to have the surgery pregnant, this also means a further wait before we can try to conceive again. With the thought, the hope, that this may be our last child-free opportunity, we go skiing in Bulgaria. I've never skied before. I have a few tries down a small slope before being asked to move on: this nursery slope is only for children staying at the hotel. So we head up to the main slope. I like the chair lift on the way up, with all that air beneath my dangling feet. I don't like hurtling down again, with the strong sense I'm about to break my neck, trying to bring my turns under control using the pizza/ French Fries method I picked up from an episode of *South Park*. This will be my last, as well as first, time skiing.

In March 2013, under local anaesthetic, it feels very weird when my eye gets to watch surgical instruments penetrate itself and prod around. My defunct lens is broken up, sucked out and replaced with an artificial lens. Since then, when I look in the mirror, I see the new lens flashing back from within. I am part bionic now.

We fall pregnant easily, but this time, there's a scepticism. We talk in terms of if not when the baby comes. I check my pants for red. But he arrives. Our son is born at 11:11 on a late November morning, his skin so soft I can hardly tell if I'm touching it or not. The time of his birth becomes a landmark on my personal map of meaning. Eight years old now, he's got used to me turning to say, 'Hey, do you know what time it is?'

More often than you might expect, it is 11:11 when I look at a clock. I am amused when I happen upon a Jon Ronson podcast episode about a community of those who also find it's very often 11:11 when they check the time. They interpret this as a sign that a great spirit guide is going to come to earth. I don't think there's anything supernatural at play. I know that when we're primed to notice something, we notice that thing more and more. I still smile, though, every time I notice it's 11:11.

I bled several times while pregnant with our daughter and it was a scary time. But she joined us safely a little over a year after our son, making this a story with a very happy ending. When I miscarried my first pregnancy, I dearly wished the outcome could have been different. But now, I look back through a different lens.

My boy said recently, as we were driving home from school, 'I wish I could be older. Mum, you and Dad should have made me as soon as you got married.'

I say, 'Remember I told you that we did try to make a baby but the baby didn't make it?'

My daughter is confused. 'Did the baby get born and then die?'

'No. The baby stopped developing and I had an operation to take it out. It's called a miscarriage. I had a miscarriage.'

They aren't sure how to feel.

I go on, 'It was sad, but,' and at this moment I look each of my children in the eye in the rearview mirror, 'I'm very happy to have the two babies that I have.'

They already know this. They know they're everything to me. The way I think of it is that if anything leading up to the conception of my children had happened differently, if that particular sperm never entered that particular egg at each of those two particular moments, I wouldn't have these children I have now. I wouldn't swap them.

22

ALISON

just because you haven't seen a unicorn…

When I reached out to parents bereaved of a baby or child, Alison got in touch saying 'I'm not sure if our experience is of any value to your research.' She and her husband had lost their 20-year-old daughter to suicide. I knew that hearing their story would be of value to me.

As Alison boils the kettle, I take in her garden, remark on the red-leaved acer tree, bright with long-beamed autumn light. Alison tells me Lara loved it – she could see it from her bedroom window – and so they didn't prune it. It is really getting too big now. Pruning acers is tricky – if you don't do it right, the tree can die – and so they've put it off.

*

Alison's daughter, Lara, died a year and a half ago. Looking back, there were signs of the OCD from when she was tiny, around five years old. She developed little rituals that seemed to reassure her, like lining up her dolls and teddies in a certain way; tapping the car before she got in and as she got out. Alison didn't know what it was at the time, but over the years the symptoms worsened; professionals began to refer to OCD traits and finally confirmed the diagnosis. By the time Lara reached 15, her OCD was so severe she could barely leave the house and she stopped eating. She believed she wasn't worthy of eating things she loved. She'd make superstitious bargains that if she ate nothing all day, nothing bad would happen. She became so ill that she was sectioned and sent to an adolescent inpatient unit. Lara believed she was entirely responsible for the safety of her family, and that if she didn't follow her elaborate rituals precisely, members of her family would die. She believed that catastrophic things would happen if she wrote the numbers 3 or 5; she took her GCSEs in hospital and managed to pass her maths exam without ever writing either of those numbers.

During her first admission to hospital, staff encouraged Lara to challenge what her OCD was telling her. Lara tried to do so and a few days later, her grandfather died. A year later, again when she was trying to challenge her OCD, her grandmother died too. So for her that was validation: *that's what happens when I don't do the rituals – someone I love dies.* It was a lot to shoulder. One day, Lara was at the very edge at Beachy Head, thinking of jumping off. She looked back along the curve of the cliff. There was a car, first in the distance, then close enough to see the driver's face. He looked directly at her, then drove over the edge. Lara believed she was innately evil; in her mind, it was looking at her, seeing her, that caused the man to die.

To see her daughter suffer like this shattered what Alison had assumed about the world. She'd been brought up by two devout Billy Graham converts, and initially, she accepted their faith. She liked the way the church wrapped up each stage of life – the christening, the wedding and the death – in a comforting ritual. Religion tells you what to do at those big moments. When, as a teenager, one of her friends died, Alison was comforted by the idea they'd be reunited in a better place. When they were small, Alison took Lara and her older sister Rachel to church in the tiny village where they lived then. It was very encompassing and welcoming and the vicar was happy for the girls to have a go reading a lesson, stumbling through the words. But when the family moved, it was to a more old-fashioned and conservative area. Alison struggled to find a church she could relate to, so she stopped going to church for a while and became more detached from her former faith. It was after Lara was first hospitalised that Alison dumped religion completely in all forms. There couldn't possibly be a God who would inflict this amount of pain on her child, and not just on her, but on the other children in the hospital. It was very hard to see these kids, some as young as 10, 11, 12, being so hurt and struggling so much. To see girls who had starved themselves to the point they could no longer walk. To see children whose soft skin was criss-crossed with scars, and whose eyes were full of shame and fear. Alison went to see the local vicar seeking answers, *how could this be?* Apparently, it was all part of God's plan, and 'Who are we to question?' But that didn't wash because a number of these children ended up dead, so what plan was it for them? Not a very good one.

It felt risky for Alison to give up her faith, because it had been a comfort blanket all her life till then. When Lara died, it would have been wonderful to have the idea that she was still living, only somewhere else, and that one day they'd be reunited. But no, she couldn't actually believe that. And besides, if she did believe there was a way they could be together once more, Alison would definitely have killed herself too.

At 17, Lara was doing really well. She'd been an inpatient for two years and was making quite a substantial recovery – on meds that suited her, challenging her OCD every day, and starting to have home visits. She was starting to live – meeting friends, going to concerts, sitting down to a meal with the family. Loads of things she hadn't been able to do before. Then of course she hit 18 and was transferred to adult services. She was moved to the local acute unit, for adults up to 65. The team wanted to start afresh, so they stopped nearly all her medication and therapy, and said, right, now that you're an adult we're going to reassess you. That was the beginning of the downward spiral, because they misdiagnosed her. And then there was a two-year battle to get her back on medication, to get her therapy that was for OCD, to get any help at all. At the point she took her life, they were just beginning to think *ok maybe we can approach this a different way*. But it was too late. Lara's OCD was the worst it had ever been, and in addition to that she had lost hope because she couldn't see there was going to be any solution, or any help coming her way. She said she couldn't fight on her own any longer – she'd done it for two years and all her strength was gone. She said, 'If this is my life, I'd rather be dead.'

In the January, she took a massive overdose and it stopped her heart. In the hospital, they gave her CPR. The consultant was very good – she kept coming in to where Alison and her husband, Greg were waiting, to tell them what was going on. 'We're doing everything we can,' and then 'We just can't get her heart started' and then 'Honestly, we might not be able to win this one, so unless we can get her heart started in the next five, ten minutes, we're just not going to manage it.' And then her heart re-started. It had been 45 minutes. After that, Lara was on life support for about a week and there was a great deal of concern about possible brain damage from being starved of oxygen. There was some damage. But it was amazing, it was stunning, the recovery she made! And they got an extra eleven weeks with her.

The problem was, she suffered short-term and long-term memory loss. Lara spent at that stage 75, 80% of her time doing rituals, and before her overdose, these had relied on her near-perfect memory. Now she was in acute distress because she knew something was wrong, but she couldn't remember what she had to do to put it right, to keep her loved ones safe. And she couldn't remember a life before the OCD, because that part of her memory had gone. She saw friends, and knew she knew them, but couldn't remember how or why. She was under Section 3 but home on leave. She stuck a note next to her pillow saying 'If you've just woken up, don't worry, it's like this every morning, you just don't remember, you take your medication at 9, this person is your friend, this is what you're meant to do, this is what you're not meant to do...' There were stickies all over her bedroom to remind her what to say and do. Her suicidal thoughts increased but there didn't seem to be much anyone could do. And then one morning she went missing.

The local police forces had been called out regarding Lara many times before. They were not as prompt as they could have been this time. When they finally found her, there was no coming back from the massive overdose she'd taken.

There is to be an Article 2 inquest, to assess whether a number of local services played a part in Lara's death by failing to protect her life. Alison would like to believe that the inquest will look into what went wrong so that it doesn't happen to anybody else, but right now that seems like just a crock of shit. The 'interested parties' have engaged the services of the top lawyer when it comes to inquests and negligence, and she just thinks *why would they do that if they've nothing to hide?* It is difficult for her to hope – unless the coroner is exceptional – that Lara's inquest will have any impact on local services at all. But if she does get lucky and is listened to, if she gets the chance to say what's important to her mind and not have it swept under the carpet, that will mean an element of peace for her and for the family. There was not one particular incident that made Lara want to die, nor one particular person whose negligence allowed it to happen. There were a whole series of people and incidences. Instead of having a team that were behind her, helping her beat the OCD, Lara had two years of being constantly told that she probably didn't have OCD, that what she had was more like borderline personality disorder. Alison and her husband did not believe that for a second. Experts who had assessed Lara were saying 'No, it's OCD,' but the community team went 'Puh, it's not *our* experts, we're not listening.' When you're up against something like that and you cannot even dent it, when the result of your inability to make an impact is that your child dies, then you think – there's got to be something we can do to change that. *If we can just get them to communicate more, to listen more...*Even if the 'interested parties' still say 'It wasn't our fault,' just going through the process maybe will help other parents think *ok, well we're not alone in this, it's really rubbish, but it happens and we're not alone.*

It is difficult for Alison, Greg, and their older daughter, Rachel, to support one another, because they are each grieving in very different ways. Rachel has busied herself with other things – making plans, getting married. At first glance, she might seem to be carrying on as normal but to anyone who looks hard enough, it will be apparent she's very fragile, and hasn't even begun to come to terms with her little sister's death. Greg looks at the photo albums for hours, but for Alison it's too hard to look at images of Lara when she isn't here. Alison has wanted to talk but Greg hasn't. He gets on his motorbike and rides around for hours, because you need that utter focus on a bike, and other thoughts get forced out. Alison can see how families don't survive a thing like this. Still, she and her husband do manage moments of quiet reflection together. They go to the local beauty spot where Lara died, to place flowers. The first year, they did it every week; this year, they've felt less compelled, but they still go once or twice a month, and there is something bonding in it.

Soon after Lara died, a friend-who-is-no-longer told Alison 'I know how you feel, my dog died.' She has had people cross the road – acquaintances who used to stop and have a chat – and that is very painful. Do they think suicide's contagious? Do they think she'll scream and rant at them? She has no idea! She has friends who tell her all about their own children. *Really? Do I want to hear how successful your kid is? My kid is dead!* Other friends think they're being helpful by not mentioning Lara's name. She tries to see it from their point of view – people don't know what to say. But that's no excuse in her book! She still has a lot of rage going on. *If you don't know what to say, say you don't know what to say! Say 'I don't know what to say.' Say 'I'm sorry, I don't know what to say.'* Sometimes in the street or at a meeting there'll be someone who tells her that 'It's God's will' or 'She's at peace', but *no, she's fucking dead!* She just can't listen to that stuff about a better place. It is hard not to hit or swear; she has to walk away instead. Alison's deeply-religious dear father died two months ago. It was difficult to talk about Lara with him, but they managed because they loved each other. He believed they would see Lara again one day, but he didn't often speak of that, because he knew where Alison stood.

There are also the ones who've really stepped up to the mark. The ones who persisted in saying 'I'm here if you want to talk' or 'Come and meet me for a coffee' or 'Can I come round?' even though Alison spent the first six months saying 'No, no, no.' The ones who came round with a stew and said 'Here's the stew, don't worry about washing up,' who didn't expect to get invited in, just 'Here's the stew' and left. The ones who let her rant when she needs to and don't try to offer solutions or logical explanations. The people who are not embarrassed when she cries. One day, Alison was standing in Sainsbury's weeping her heart out. Other people were staring but so what? Alison's friend focused only on her: 'What's wrong?' 'I can't remember what pasta she liked!' When Lara died, she'd been living on pasta and coffee, and she was very particular about the pasta because it couldn't have egg in it. In that moment, it was enormously distressing for Alison that she'd forgotten what the right type of pasta was. Some weeks later, she remembered. It was Fusilli, 500g.

At the time of Lara's death, Alison had been seeing a therapist for more than five years, because when Lara first became ill, Alison found it really difficult to deal with. The therapist helped her very much through that journey. Being able to talk to someone who is not involved in any way is an enormous help. If you talk to family, they've got their own emotions; if you talk to friends, they worry about you and may want to pacify or fix you, whereas someone unconnected can just listen. Unfortunately, Alison's therapist has moved away now. She tried to find another: she's telling her story to this person, and the therapist starts to cry. Alison's thinking, *there are people worse off than me, people who've lost more than one child.* How can you trust or offload onto a therapist who can't contain their own emotion? So that was no use.

Other parents of troubled children have been the most support. It's just the shorthand of knowing, understanding, no explanations needed. She's stayed in contact with some of the families who had kids at the same inpatient unit as Lara. Alison has tried support groups. Compassionate Friends is for parents who have lost a child by any means and SOBS is for people who have lost loved ones through suicide. Neither hit the spot for Alison. Because if you've lost a child to cancer, that's a different journey and a different loss. And if you've lost your terminally ill grandfather to suicide, that's not the same as losing your child. On Twitter, though, Alison finds community. Other bereaved parents; other people who've been through inquests; or just other people who like cats. Alison will check in on Twitter, usually each morning, definitely each night before she goes to bed.

Alison is just beginning to separate out the good memories of Lara from all the pain. It is difficult, because to find the truly happy times, she has to go way back. Lara was a gorgeous little girl – and that's not just mother-blindness speaking! She had a very open nature; she was curious and the kindest soul ever. The one who didn't want to stand on ants.

'There's an ant, Mama!'

'Yes, there's thousands of ants!'

'Yeah, but to that ant it's important!'

She was a vegetarian and then a vegan. It makes Alison proud to think how Lara and her friend were the first inpatients on the adolescent unit to think of doing something to help others with mental health problems, by raising funds for Mind. They did a sponsored star jump that raised £4723. She loved swimming. She was really interested in how things work. It makes Alison smile to remember Lara's ingenuity, how she challenged staff at the hospital where she was an inpatient. They had a keypad on the door as security – Lara cracked the code in 90 minutes. They switched to swipe cards and she got very good at picking people's pockets. Again, they changed their system. Then she worked out that the clasp on her bracelet could be used to pick the lock. They had to put out a nationwide bulletin saying, 'Girls who've got these bracelets – they can open the doors!'

On all of these occasions, Lara was trying to get home. The adolescent unit was some 80, 90 miles away and yet Lara once managed to get out very late at night and made it home. She would have had to walk four or five miles to the local station, change at another hub, and then walk again, and she did all that, with no shoes, no money, that's how determined she was. And she's still at home. Her ashes are. For the first year, Alison found it very difficult to leave the house. They still can't go on holiday for any length of time because she needs to get back. There is this illogical desire to still be close to Lara, even though she isn't *really* here. Her room is still the same – the only difference is that Alison has closed the bedroom door to maintain Lara's smell. Alison dusts the room but cannot move things. Because Lara believed herself inherently evil, she did not allow family members within about four feet of her for their own safety. While Lara was alive, Alison was never allowed to set foot in her bedroom. So at first, to go in there seemed a betrayal, but now it's a connection to her. When Lara died, Alison had five years' worth of hugs to squeeze into five hours with her daughter's body.

Little glimmers of happy moments sometimes do come through to Alison. Swimming together in the sea as a family, on the last holiday they were able to have together. The conversations they'd have in the car. Because Lara couldn't drive, Alison used to drive her everywhere, and although the conversations they had were often incredibly difficult, that time together was important. The day before she died, they were driving up along the ridge where you get these glorious views. Alison said, 'Lara, look at that fabulous sunset!' and at the same time, they both said 'Look at the clouds!' Because the colours were wonderful. And Lara laughed, 'You always talk about the frigging clouds!'

Lara's friends remember her, too. It was enormously important to her to be a supportive friend. Generally, you're not allowed your smartphone at an inpatient unit, so texts and online messaging were out of the question, and Lara would not speak on the communal phone, so she and the other girls had stacks of letters. Lara was always writing what you might call 'good hope' letters, and positivity books for her friends, to give them something to refer to when they were struggling. She wrote 'I believe you can,' 'Stay strong,' 'Don't quit;' she sent a biro drawing of a rainbow with 'HAPPINESS!!!!' written along its curve; she wrote 'You said last week was quite tough and so I just wanted to let you know how awesome you are.xxxxx' She sent a notebook and on the first page told her friend to 'Fill this book with positive memories, quotes, items and comments for when you are feeling a little down or struggling so it can pick you up and make you feel better.' Some of Lara's friends from her adolescent unit days stay in touch with Alison. A few are still quite ill, but others are getting on with their lives. In a way, that's difficult for Alison to hear about, yet in another way it's lovely. They tell Alison how they re-read Lara's letters and get a very strong sense of her coming through, how when the tough times come, Lara's words of advice and support can lift them up still. One friend tells how she can almost hear Lara take the piss when she puts Ed Sheeran on, but says, 'I'm gonna play it anyway!'

Lara's funeral service was beautiful. The place was covered in glitter – how they cleared it up afterwards, Alison will never know. Friends and family painted huge butterflies and stuck them up all over the room. There was a tree on which each person hung a little origami butterfly. The celebrant brought a basket of those little tubes of bubble blowers, so during the service people were blowing bubbles. Though Lara had been brought up going to church, she grew to hate organised religion, believing it responsible for a lot of what is wrong in the world – the wars and the intolerance. She had expressed that she wanted nothing connected with religion at her funeral, so they removed the cross from the wall and in its place hung a huge purple unicorn head. There were unicorns, too, dancing around the bottom of the coffin. Lara used to say, 'Just because you haven't seen one, doesn't mean they don't exist. Most people haven't seen me, but I exist!'

She exists. That text circulating the internet, 'Why You Want A Physicist To Speak At Your Funeral,' had resonance for Greg. It refers to the first law of thermodynamics: that 'No energy gets created in the universe and none destroyed.' For Greg, it helped to remember that Lara's energy hasn't died, that not a bit of her is gone from our universe, she is just 'less orderly.' For Alison, something that's raised a smile is hearing about the studies showing that cells of a foetus can stay in the mother's body for the rest of her life. In her brain, her bones, her liver, lungs and blood. It is a phenomenon known as fetomaternal microchimerism. How incredibly amazing to think that not only is Lara a part of her metaphorical heart, but that on a cellular level, she could carry her child within her still.

For the first months, Alison couldn't concentrate long enough to finish anything book-length, and it is still hard, but she's beginning to read some things that other people have written about their losses, and reading these accounts makes it all less alien. She had bought into that idea of the five stages of grief – denial, anger, bargaining, depression and acceptance, then you're done and dusted. Of course, the reality is much less neat. Reading about bereavement – books like *I Wasn't Ready to Say Goodbye* – has helped her understand her feelings better. And she got a lot from Sara Ryan's book about the death of her son, Connor Sparrowhawk, because this was another mother who had been through something similar.

Because the support groups on offer in the area didn't quite fit her situation, Alison's had the idea to set up a group herself, for parents bereaved by suicide. She's got the literature ready, and a venue set up. She's spoken to people she thinks will help publicise it. She's about to attend a training day to gain a bit more confidence with running stuff like that. Once the inquest is over, she hopes to start the group up. It may help someone. Apart from this, she and Greg want to help other children in the ways that Lara couldn't get help. It is common for people who are having a mental health crisis, that the hours between 1 and 4 am are a particularly difficult time. Apart from A & E, there's nowhere for people to go. They're looking at offering a crisis service that runs all night long, for 16 to 26-year-olds. Somewhere these kids can just walk in and know they'll have someone to talk to. They're starting to fundraise towards what they're calling Lara's Project. Alison would like to think that they can help people in future. It seems meaningless, in a way, to speak of hopes for the future. The future that she hoped for is dead and gone before it had a chance to be. She used to admire her mother-in-law's dining table – it could fit 20 people around it, no problem. She had an image of all of them around it – Greg's parents and her own, her brother and his family, the kids and their boyfriends or husbands. When her mother-in-law died, the table came to Alison, but now there's just the three of them in the house, they rarely use it. Perhaps, if Rachel has babies, they'll bring a future in which Alison could once again invest hope. She likes to think so.

This year is a little better than last year. Sometimes, Alison can think of Lara without dissolving into a puddle of weeping hysteria. Sometimes she manages to go for Sunday lunch at the pub. If it's a good day, she may even get down to the beach, for a swim or just to sit. When things are really bad, she can't get out of bed, can't wash or dress, and doesn't eat properly. (When Lara died, Alison thought *at least I'll lose weight now! Skinny in grief!* But no, her grief is the comfort-eating kind, the kind that heavily relies on chocolate.) This year, when she can feel she's getting too low, she's got a little better at making a concerted effort to have a coffee with a friend or go for a walk. These are her two main lifters. She likes to walk where there are lots of trees and not too many people. This area is blessed with lots of trees. Alison sometimes walks in the woods nearby, where the grandeur of the oaks and beeches fills her with a sense of her place in the universe. There is comfort in the reliable rhythms and renewals of nature, in the promise that even when the leaves are blackening underfoot, spring is always on its way again.

*

I was nervous about meeting Alison. Lara's death was still an open wound and not a scar she had learned to live with. I didn't want to make things worse. I felt it was important that, even though I knew the story I would hear would be very sad, I should control my own emotions. I wanted to leave the space for Alison to tell me about losing Lara. I talked about myself and my own children only so far as to answer Alison's questions.

So I didn't say at the time that on mornings when the sun is evaporating rain from pavements, on our walk to school, the kids and I move stranded worms to the undergrowth so they won't get trampled or dry out, though the radio tells me there are around a million worms in an acre of land. It matters to that worm. It matters to that ant. I'm with Lara on this. And I think about her often.

23

IN OUR HEARTS AND IN THE WORLD

'Two facts – that the dead once lived; and that one loved them and mourned their loss – are inexpungeably a part of the world's history. So the presence of those who lived can never be removed from time, which is to say there is a kind of eternity after all.'

A.C. Grayling, *The Meaning of Things*

When a loved one dies, life can feel rudderless. Some grievers find that carrying out rituals brings some order to the chaos and helps hold the loved one close. When we think of rituals, we may think first of ceremonies and traditions of a religious nature. But a recent study found only 5% of the rituals engaged in by bereaved participants were religious. Instead, most rituals were a unique reflection of the bond between the griever and their lost loved one. We can all find our own ways to affirm our continuing connection to a loved one who has died. We can create space and time for remembrance each week, on anniversary days, or whenever feels right. Alison and Greg find some solace in going together to lay flowers at the beauty spot where their daughter died. Arthur and Wendy honour their son Ian's memory by raising a glass of one of his favourite brews and listening to his music. We may choose to wear something that belonged to our loved one, assemble a photo album or cook their favourite meal.

Though non-religious grievers may not believe our lost loved one is looking down on us or listening to our words, some find it helpful to continue communicating with a loved one who has died. Particularly when someone has died suddenly or too young, we may feel stuck with undelivered communications and need to find ways to continue to express our love. Surviving bereavement is about doing whatever helps, even if it may not seem rational. Bob will sometimes call one of his sons when he visits his wife Vera's grave, as a way of keeping her up to date with family news. Kim speaks to her baby and her best friend when she goes to tend their graves.

Our loved ones live in our hearts symbolically. We may also find comfort in the thought of our loved ones being with us still in more literal, physical ways. A friend told me he is consoled by the idea that when he drinks a glass of water, it contains atoms which may previously have passed through the bodies of his mother and grandmother. We may like the fact we are carrying our parents' genes into the future. Alison likes the thought that, through the phenomenon of microchimerism, a small number of Lara's cells may be present in her own internal organs, a legacy from the months that Lara grew inside her. Her husband, Greg, found value in radio journalist Aaron Freeman's assurance that 'no energy gets created in the universe and none is destroyed,' in the thought that every particle that was Lara, still exists.

When a child or young adult dies, they will certainly have made a mark upon their parents, but it can feel so very wrong they didn't get fair chance to make their mark upon the world. Non-religious parents don't believe their child has grown angel wings or is being looked after by Grandma; there will be no compensation for the child's unlived life in a world beyond. Yet, bereaved parents often find some sense of meaning and consolation through creating a legacy for their child. It is often important for parents that the world should be a better place because their child existed; they work to make it so. When Lara died, it boosted Alison to hear that her daughter's positive messages had helped her friends, in their struggles with their own mental health. Arthur, too, was uplifted to read, on the Facebook tribute pages set up for Ian, how much his son meant to his friends. But both Alison and Arthur wanted to see their child's life and death making bigger changes in the world. Alison hopes that the work she is putting into Lara's inquest will help prevent future tragedies, and that setting up a local group for parents bereaved by suicide can soften the pain of others who are going through a similar loss. She and her husband Greg are raising funds in their daughter's memory, so that other vulnerable young people will be better supported in future. Arthur and Wendy have also raised money in Ian's name; their efforts have meant many others suffering from blood and bone cancers have been able to enjoy their time away from hospital, making memories to treasure. Arthur is still finding new ways to send out messages to the future, so that people will know about his son, Ian.

When a baby or very young child dies, the urge can be especially strong for parents to let the world know their child existed. Bereaved parents are still parents. Like other parents, they feel joy and pride at having created another person. Helping a child to make a mark on the world can feel like a way of continuing to parent. Some like to write her name in the sand when they visit the coast, or show his picture and have people say they'd like to smush his cheeks. The efforts of bereaved parents to raise money or awareness can keep their child present for other people. It can mean a lot to hear a loved child's name on another person's lips, especially given that there remains something of a taboo around child loss. In the Sands Garden at the National Memorial Arboretum in Staffordshire, the paths are lined with hundreds of small stones on which parents have written their baby's name, or a short message, in indelible ink. After May died, Kim found some solace through helping to train medical staff in how to deal with parents who are losing a baby. Thanks to Kim's efforts to raise funds for a side room, parents whose baby can't live can have a gentler experience now, at the hospital where May was born. I hope that Lara, Ian and May's parents will feel that this book is also a part of their child's ongoing legacy.

24

SOPHIE

going through the big stuff young

For some who shared their stories with me, several decades had gone by since their loved ones died. Sophie and Alan were able to tell me how their grief had changed with time, as well as how living through loss had changed them.

*

Sophie was six when her mum died of cancer, following an illness of two or three years. During these years, Sophie recalls sleepovers of a week or so with friends and neighbours, which must have been when her mum was having treatment. The diagnosis was terminal; the chemo and radiotherapy were to give her mum a bit more time. Sophie was sent to a 'talking doctor,' who, through play, art and talking, tried to prepare this little girl for what was coming. She came to understand that her mother would die, and that death was final. What she remembers most of her visits to the talking doctor is that he had one of those old-fashioned telephones you can pull along on a piece of string.

Sophie went to her mum's funeral; she has been told that her mum wanted it to be an upbeat day, a celebration of her life. Sophie has a snapshot image from that day of skipping with her best friend Eva, and the other kids who lived on the little cul-de-sac where no cars drove and it was safe to play out on the road. Everyone brought presents for little Sophie – a pen that was also a torch, a Sony Walkman – and when she went to stay with an aunt, she'd get free access to the sweet tin.

Sophie's parents had split before she turned a year old. For her first six years, she'd lived with her mum in Holland. Her English father had been like Santa, turning up once a year or so with gifts. During her mum's illness, Sophie's dad moved to Holland, and formed a new relationship. So, it was with her father and her stepmother that Sophie moved in after her mum died. It was not a good relationship, however; Sophie would come downstairs after bedtime and ask if they could argue more quietly so she could sleep. After a year, her step mum kicked her dad out, and Sophie had to go too. They were slightly homeless in the way that happens when a relationship breaks down. Her dad took her back to England. Lost for what to do with this seven-year-old motherless girl, he thought the best way to give her some stability while he sorted himself out was to put her in a boarding school. He never did seem to sort himself out and she remained at boarding school till 18.

At school, there was chapel every morning, hymns and sermons every day. When Sophie got upset about her mum, the teachers would say 'She's looking down on you from heaven' or 'Your mum is in a better place.' Sophie knew her mum wasn't up there on a fluffy cloud – her mum was dead and gone, full stop. As an adult, she believes it's best to listen to a child and say you've heard their feelings. At the time, though, she knew the teachers were well-meaning, trying to show her love in their own way. Sophie's own daughter is now eight. She can't imagine saying 'Goodbye darling, I'll see you at half term.' Lying in a dorm with five or six other boarders is a very different thing from going home and snuggling with your family. In the summer holidays, Sophie used to spend a couple of weeks with her mum's best friend, a couple of weeks with one, and a couple with another aunt, a week or so with her dad and that would be the holiday done. They held different views on how she should be parented and would each try to influence her in their slot of time.

Sophie was a troubled teenager. She started smoking at 14, stopped trying hard in lessons, and drank a lot, sometimes to the point of losing consciousness. She was angry at the world and didn't like herself much. She felt alone, the odd one out. One of her friends would argue on the phone with their mother, hang up and say 'I wish she'd die!' When meeting new

126

people, Sophie became wary of telling them about her mum, because there'd be an awkward pause in conversation, and she'd get treated differently when people knew. One of her teachers gave her a book called *Motherless Daughters*, which she read with tears streaming because it resonated deeply. She read that children who lose their mothers in middle childhood can have the hardest time coping because they're cognitively advanced enough to grasp the depth of loss, but haven't yet mastered the management of their emotions. Reading the stories of other women who'd lost their mothers young was greatly comforting for Sophie: that sense of *oh, these feelings I have are not unique to me, lots of people have them.*

Sophie's dad never spoke about her mum. If you ask questions but get no satisfactory answers, you learn to avoid that subject. Sophie's memories of her mum are mainly of fleeting moments in which her mum in fact is a kind of secondary character. Being in a hospital room, with her mum somewhere behind her, lying in bed probably – but that is her mind filling in a blank, because what Sophie actually recalls is looking out of the window at rabbits playing on the grass. If she casts her mind back further, there are snippets of days out – digging in a sand pit or splashing in a pool; again, her mother's presence in these scenes is almost incidental. She can picture the layout of the living room in the home she shared with her mum, but Sophie cannot recall the sound of her mum's laugh. In some of the photos she has of her mum, her hair is curly, but in others it is straight, and Sophie doesn't know its natural state. Did her mum have it permed or did she straighten her hair?

Sophie's aunts – her mum's sisters – told her some things, but only the good stuff and the funny little stories. She used to like to hear what her mum got up to as a child; how, when she was eight or nine she had an operation on her ear. She never used to play with dolls much, but was given one to comfort her in hospital. Everyone would comment 'She really loves that doll – she takes it with her everywhere!' The truth was she hated the hospital food and had learnt she could rip the doll's head off, fill it with yucky stuff, then take it to the toilet and flush everything away. Such anecdotes let Sophie catch little wisps of her mother as a person. But she'll never know her mother in the round – her political leanings, how she felt about being a single mum, how she juggled her career as a doctor, who she truly was.

Sophie has no felt memory of her mother's love for her. She is told she was her mum's world and that is kind of reassuring. It is at life's milestones that Sophie has sometimes felt her mother's absence sharply, grieved the life that could have been. Each Mother's Day at school, she'd make a card for her mum's best friend, or one of her aunts. When her daughter was born, she would have liked to ask her mum how she'd found that newborn stage. She'd like to know what her mum would have thought of her husband and her kids. There can be no answers to these questions.

A notebook of her mum's words opens a little window on the six years the two of them had together. 'Today it rained and you were not happy at all. You were very cross with me when I said I couldn't make it stop.' 'This morning you woke me up and proudly presented me with a cup of coffee, which I gratefully drank down. It was water from the cold tap, mixed with granules.' 'This is the four-leaf clover which we found on our walk today!' 'I left the room for five minutes. When I came back in you denied all knowledge of the little piles of snipped blond hair.' It is something-better-than-nothing to have her mother's words.

As a child, Sophie was very loyal to her father, though other adults sometimes criticised him. As she grew up, his faults were more apparent and Sophie's love was less blinkered; their relationship wasn't great, but it was ok. During her uni years, she'd visit him once a month, a two-and-a-half-hour train ride away. His kidney function was decreasing over time, though not to the point of needing dialysis. One day, Sophie got a call to say he'd had a heart attack and was in hospital. She set out to see him and on the train she got a second call.

When she explained that she was on her way, they said 'Ok, we'll speak to you when you get here.'

'How serious is it?'

'We'll speak to you when you get here.'

When she got there, a nurse took her to a private room and told her that her father had died. It was a shock. Sophie could have caught an earlier train, but it hadn't sounded urgent. Instead, she'd had a cup of tea at home and waited till after morning rush hour, when the trains got cheaper.

Sophie was a 23-year-old orphan. A couple of months previously, she had split up with her uni boyfriend, but now she called him up and begged him to come to the funeral with her, and, amazingly, he did. She needed someone to support her that day and he did it perfectly. After the funeral, they briefly got back together, but the reasons for the break-up were still there, so it couldn't last. Sophie is forever grateful, though, that he was kind enough to put aside all bitterness and be there for her when she needed him. Sophie took some time off work and sat in the park, looking at the trees, not thinking about anything. She existed in a small bubble of simple things – showering, sitting with a friend, a bit of basic housework in the flat she lived in by herself. Sometimes she'd sob for hours, submerged by waves of not so much *I miss my dad* but more *I'm all alone now.* After a couple of months, some friends were thinking *what, you're still not over it?* But others were there if she wanted to phone up and cry; they were there still if she didn't answer her phone for weeks at a time. They loved her.

She went back to work and began to manically date, looking for fun and distraction. At one point she was having weekly dates with four different blokes, and then she met Ben. She told him she was nowhere near available for any kind of relationship and couldn't take on the burden of anyone else's feelings or expectations at that time. Ben had just come out of a long-term relationship himself and said he wasn't looking for anything serious either, so Sophie granted him a spot on her dating rota. Over time, the other dates fizzled out, but Ben remained. Christmas came, and Sophie wanted to spend the day ugly-crying by herself. Several friends invited her to spend Christmas with their families and Ben did too, but she turned them all down. On Christmas morning, he rang and asked if he could drop round presents for Sophie, then he took her out for ice cream at the only open café in town. He went off for his family Christmas in the afternoon. It was only the following year Sophie realised he'd willingly given up half his Christmas day to make sure she'd spend at least some of hers smiling and eating ice cream. Things progressed at Sophie's pace and two years later she moved in with Ben; after a couple more they had Amelia.

Sophie's first thought on discovering she was pregnant wasn't to decorate the baby's room or buy tiny clothes. It was to make a will. People say things like 'I could get hit by a bus tomorrow' but they don't truly believe that. Sophie knows the kind of thing that really can happen, because she's lived it. She wanted to know whatever happened to her, the baby would be taken care of. She doesn't have the luxury of assuming her world is a safe place. But maybe her happiness is the flip side of that same coin. She's married to a man she loves, who loves her. She isn't thinking about a bigger house or a better job. She's not restless to chase rainbows.

Now Amelia is eight and Jacob, four. When the kids were born, Sophie's whole Dutch family flew over to meet the newborn. When they moved into their new house, the extended family came back to look around. Sometimes, there are dramas at the school gates – one mum unfriends another on Facebook, or someone's life is ruined when their car breaks down. Sophie stays out of it and doesn't sweat the small stuff. Because she's been through the big stuff and come out the other side. When she came into her mid-thirties, it hit her how hard it must have been for her mum to know she was dying, that she would go and leave her child behind. Sophie had a sense on some level that she had a hereditary expiration date. Any twinge or pain would make her think *is this the cancer coming for me now?* Now she is 37, the age her mother was when she died. But Sophie is in good health and it seems she can be confident of seeing 38, of existing longer than her mother ever did. She feels a self-assurance in trusting the resilience that has brought her this far.

Sophie doesn't talk to the kids much about her mum and dad. They know her parents are dead, but haven't asked much and she wouldn't have much to tell them anyway. But she has continued the tradition of having a little book of funny things herself. So that the children will be able to read about the things they said and did when they were small. When Sophie takes the book out to write a new entry, sometimes she looks back at pages from their younger years: 'Your beautiful sayings so far – "let's play hide and sick!" "Mummy, you have a spot…like a leopard!" "I can't go to sleep, I've forgotten how to close my eyes."' Sometimes Sophie looks back; mostly, she just enjoys each day.

25

ALAN

the expert widower

Sometimes Alan ponders different life forms. There are internal parasites which are nothing more than a blob of tissue given over to reproductive apparatus. They have no sensory organs, no mouth, no alimentary canal, no excretory apparatus. It's all provided by the host and simple diffusion. No venturing into the moonlight and smelling the night scents, no enjoying orchestral concerts for them. They simply manufacture offspring.

Alan and Susan enjoyed 25 wonderful years together and raised two great kids, before, at the age of 47, she was diagnosed with breast cancer and, after two years of worry, hope, and hopes dashed, she died aged 49. Alan was 51, and their two children were 20 and 18. Baking the cake for Amanda's 21st was one of the last things her mother did.

Alan never wavered in his atheist views during Sue's illness – he never prayed; he did, though, superstitiously park in the exact same spot each time he took her into hospital for radio. Of course, that had no impact on the outcome. The cancer spread to her chest and brain. She was given a few months to live. In fact, a month from then she'd gone. Sue and Alan were in bed when she began making noises, unable to speak properly. He called an ambulance, which came, but was not carrying any oxygen. They had adrenaline, but the ambulance man didn't know how to open the ampoule, he'd not been trained. Alan did know and said, 'Give it to me, I'll do it.'

And he did, but she was gone – there was a blood clot in her lungs. It was horrible to lose her, yet Alan knew enough to know if she'd lived longer, she might have been in for something far worse.

Amanda and Jeremy had no prior experience with death, so Alan tried to guide them. He knew it was important to let grief happen and not try to suppress it. So he told them each in turn to go up to the bedroom, lay their head on their mother's chest and tell her whatever they wanted.

They got condolence cards of course. The printed messages were useless – 'with deepest sympathy…' 'your sad loss…' Anything that spoke of Susan as a person was a comfort. People don't know what to say, but if they just say *something*…One card had a scribbled note saying, 'I always thought what lovely hair Sue had,' and Alan liked that. He noticed that people began avoiding him. Not the next-door neighbours, but people further up the street that Sue used to stop and chat to. Alan would see them cross the road so they wouldn't have to speak to him.

Four years or so after Susan died, Alan got a call out of the blue from the bereavement charity Cruse. At their training sessions for volunteers they always had a widow and a widower to come along and talk about how they'd coped. Their widower had remarried, so would Alan be willing to take his place? For example, they suggested, if Alan hadn't been able to cook, how did he learn? Where did he go to do his shopping and get his washing done? These were the things the other chap had spoken of. The widow similarly – she'd had to learn to deal with fuses and tap washers. Alan, instead, thought he would use his diary from that time to tell the audience how those first few months felt after losing Sue. He'd been given a few bereavement books by friends and in the early days had found it helpful to read other people's stories of loss, to know that what he was feeling was what other people feel as well. Maybe his journey through grief could point the way ahead for others who were just beginning theirs. He'd written a lot in that first year; he felt better after getting down on paper all those swirling thoughts. There was his diary, and also letters. When someone writes a letter of condolence, you are not expected to write back, but he did, and he kept copies. He'd just give the people at Cruse the highlights, if you can call them that.

How, on the hot June day of the funeral, he was so taken aback by the depth of the hole when they'd lowered the little casket of her ashes down into it. It was as if they were shutting her too far away. He dropped a single red rose clipped from their garden, choking at the image of his wife, two years back, choosing the bush from the catalogue. She'd watched it grow, enjoyed its colour and perfume, without thinking one day this flower would be dropped on her own grave. He'd been told writing a letter when a loved one dies might help, so he told the kids that too, and the three of them dropped a letter each into the grave. In fact he thinks it *did* help in some way. Not that she was going to read his letter, but perhaps writing down then letting go the words in some way lessened that sense of the marriage being unfinished. We're human and must do whatever we find meaningful. And in those first weeks, months, that first year, you've got to manage by whatever means you can, even if it seems illogical.

Those first weeks, his mind tried to protect him from the fact of death's finality. Despite all the evidence of Sue's death – the letters, flowers, funeral and legal arrangements – Alan was sustained by a sense that if he could only grit his teeth and hang on, he'd eventually wake to find Sue laughing kindly, 'That must have been an awful dream!' He kept a picture of her by his bedside where he'd see it first thing each day. Some of Sue's outer garments his sister took to the charity shop; some of her underclothes he burned early on and it was very painful indeed but felt like good sense, since he feared he'd never get rid of them if he didn't do it straight away. But he kept one of the nightdresses, a nice silky one. He kept it in bed at night with him, cuddled and breathed it in as if it were a favourite teddy bear. On Sue's birthday, in September, he felt he wanted to do something for her, but she was dead, and what can you do? He thought at least he could put flowers on her grave. He went to the florist and the lady said, 'Some lucky person will be very pleased with these.' Alan couldn't even answer.

He learned a lot in those first months. The sadness, loneliness and depression he had expected, but he hadn't seen the fear coming – fear of whether he could cope, of breaking down in public, unnameable terrors. And there was insomnia, loss of appetite, an inability to concentrate on anything. All of these problems would have been bad enough with Sue there to provide support, but of course she wasn't there. He felt like a hunted fox, with all its bolt holes blocked. Nothing he tried offered an escape from pain. Music was too moving, he couldn't look at photo albums. He didn't dare try alcohol. When she'd been ill and frightened and needed Alan, his tender feelings for Sue had intensified. When she died, his emotions were as fervid as back when they first met. He wandered around sighing and muttering terms of endearment like he did as a young thing. Only then, he was looking forward to a future with her, but now, he had to aim at gradually loosening the threads that bound them.

He had to try to function normally. He was a senior scientist at that time, in charge of a group of other scientists and technicians working on drug research. Things had piled up while he was away, and his boss made no allowances. Seven weeks after Sue's death, when Alan mentioned he'd been weeping for her, his boss seemed very surprised: 'She's still that close is she?' Much of the time Alan *could* function. He'd be walking along putting on a brave face, he'd take this step and be ok, but with the next one it would hit him and suddenly he'd be sobbing in the street. He'd be sitting in the evening at a friend's house, thinking *it's getting dark and I should really get back* till it occurred to him there was no one to get back to, he could stay all night if necessary. A terrible freedom. Desolation. He'd be out with his brother and his brother's wife, amazed at how they walked several steps apart. He'd dream of Susan helping him to fold up bed clothes and think *how nice to have her by my side, I wonder why we don't do this more often.* Two months after she died, it was a knife to him to see the cashier in the bank strike Sue's name from their joint account. Five months after she died comes the first diary entry in which Sue isn't mentioned. The entry speaks of things he has to do, problems at work.

Alan had returned to work grim-faced and quiet. After an awkward initial couple of weeks, most of the staff stopped saying 'Good morning' to him, as if he were somehow *persona non grata*. This made him even more grim-faced and quiet. He did not attend the Christmas party and drank his coffee in his office. Looking back, he thinks they saw a lack of feeling in his straight lips and thought him coldly-unaffected by his wife's death. They didn't know that most days he walked smartly to his office armed with a towel, wept and dried his face, and soberly continued with his work.

Joining a group for widows and widowers brought a more positive focus to his life. Mutual support amongst people who've been there, who *are* there with you. Simple companionship – a chat around a table, a few announcements, a cup of tea, perhaps a game of darts and then home. In time, Alan felt something of an expert widower and that he could have some useful input with new members. He was the recruiting officer for the group and when someone rang and said they were interested, he'd collect them for their first meeting, take them down and introduce them. There were always far more women than men in the group, so if the new member was a man, he sometimes needed a bit of extra help. What Alan would find is that he'd get the man sat down with a few others, but if he then went off to do something else, he'd look back and see the new bloke sitting staring at the ceiling and the women talking quietly to each other. So Alan would go and sit with him, ease him into the conversation that way. It seemed to Alan that a woman didn't want to be seen talking to a man in case the other ladies thought she was after him. A few of the women were saying how they hated Sundays – they'd always cooked a meal for their husbands, but now, what was the point? So Alan said, 'Well look, there's three of you in the same position. Why don't you two invite these two to lunch next Sunday, then you invite them the following Sunday, and so on?' And they did.

When people first came to the group, often they didn't want to talk about their grief. They were looking for diversion, living in a little envelope of the present. Alan organised trips to concerts, walks in the countryside. A lot of the members, not being country folk, weren't used to walking in the woods. Alan would take along a magnifying glass, share with the others the loveliness of bluebell frills up close.

Now he's been 34 years without Sue. The first 13 he was alone (how quick to write, how long to live through.) Then he found happiness again with Alina. He is 85 now, and in reasonable health. His brain still works, though his knees are getting wobbly. You don't choose to be a person, he reflects. You could have been a malarial parasite. How wonderful to be a human being! A creature that can experience the world, that can know love.

26

THE NATURE PRESCRIPTION

The picture of widows and widowers gathering round to see bluebells through a magnifying glass has stayed with me. Many of us feel some sense of enlargement and enrichment when we immerse ourselves in nature. Recent studies appear to confirm what we intuitively sense – that people who are more connected to nature are happier.

More than 50% of people now live in urban areas, a trend which is on the increase, and which is associated with rising levels of mental illness, including depression. A growing body of research indicates that 'the nature prescription' can benefit our mental well-being in a range of ways. Going for a walk reduces stress and anxiety; these benefits are augmented when we walk in a natural rather than an urban environment. Walking in a forest, for example, has been shown to have a significantly greater positive impact on cardiovascular relaxation, in comparison with walking in a city centre. High levels of activity in the subgenual prefrontal cortex are linked to risk of mental illness, including depression; when we walk in nature, activity in this region of our brains quietens down, and we focus less on negative emotions such as guilt and remorse. Studies show that people find blue spaces even more restorative than green ones. Water reflects light, creates relaxing sounds, and offers potential for immersion in literal and metaphorical ways. When we're walking on a beach, next to a river or in woodland, our focus turns toward our natural environment, in a way that can help our troubles feel less overwhelming.

The world still looked pretty bleak to Alison when she spoke to me 18 months after her daughter took her own life, but she told me that being in nature was one of the few things that could lift her up. She was able to find solace walking in the nearby woods where the grand, towering trees offer some sense of security, some sense that life endures. On good days, she gets down to the sea to have a swim or watch the waves. Bob finds comfort in noticing how each week the annual cycle of flowers around Vera's grave rolls beautifully onwards – with snowdrops followed by primroses and cowslips. Many bereaved people like Alison, Bob and Alan, find solace in the natural world. Often there is a feeling of surprise that the beauty of nature continues after a loved one's death, and that this beauty can still delight and bring joy. Trees standing side by side offer a kind of company without making any demands. There is no requirement to answer questions or make polite conversation. Wide open spaces can help to take us out of our small selves. It can be restorative to feel we're all part of some bigger, enduring thing.

27

DIANA AND BRIDGET

and good that comes from loss

Diana had a tough time towards the end of her husband's life. Laurence had Alzheimer's for his last 7 years. For much of that time Diana cared for him at home, but when she was diagnosed with cancer and needed chemo, she had to put Laurence in a care home. Around that time, Diana got into a terrible crash while cycling and was incapacitated for a long while. Then, it was very sad when she lost her lovely husband. She had been losing him for years though, and as well as sadness there was relief, for him and for herself.

Diana used to play violin in a string quartet, but she broke her elbow badly in the crash, and was no longer able to turn her hand enough to reach the positions needed.

She went to see a physiotherapist who promised 'I'm going to get you back to playing.'

After a number of sessions, Diana said, 'I thought the NHS were limiting everything – isn't there someone saying that woman's had quite enough?'

But the physio said 'I decide who I'm going to work with,' and she held onto hope when Diana was feeling very discouraged.

With this brilliant person's help, Diana was able to play again. It is something she thought she'd lost, but has, still. The quartet was invited to the Christmas do at the nearby anthropological museum, where they sat and played amidst the shrunken heads. No one really listened, because they were too busy drinking champagne and chatting, and that was fine with Diana. The quartet aren't good enough to do a proper concert, but they can play well enough to move themselves, and that is lovely.

Soon after Laurence died, Diana sold the family home and moved into a retirement apartment. She doesn't have to deal with stairs or gardening now, and finds she likes living alone, yet knowing there's a community of people living around her. She can't cycle any more, but she's discovered walking – because she never used to walk – and she absolutely loves it.

*

When Bridget's husband died, a woman came and knocked on the door and asked if she would like to go to the bereavement group at the village church. Bridget said 'No thanks.' Several people suggested to her 'This is where you must miss having religion,' and she told them 'I know you can't understand it, but no, not in the least.' After her husband, Jack, had a stroke at the age of 53, Bridget nursed him 24 hours a day, seven days a week for 12 years. When he died, she took the line *he's dead, I'm alive, staying at home thinking of what might have been isn't going to bring him back, if it would, I'd be there. But he's not coming back.*

She hadn't been able to travel for many years. She joined the Commonwealth Magistrates' and Judges' Association because she realised their conferences would offer a good opportunity to travel with a group of people. They'd all be on their own too, as spouses didn't attend. That first year, there were trips to Singapore and Malaysia – trips packed full of seeing, learning, and exploring. Bridget didn't want to go back somewhere she'd been before with Jack. She didn't want to sit on the beach picturing him windsurfing out there, yelling at her 'Come on in, it's lovely!' Instead, what got her through that time was taking on a programme that was going to be quite demanding: visits to courts and prisons, followed by formal dinners at which she was called upon to give several speeches and presentations. Bridget found the whole experience exhausting but exhilarating. She saw that after caring, after being widowed, there was a route to taking part in life again.

*

Psychologists Richard Tedeschi and Lawrence Calhoun coined the term posttraumatic growth, which they define as 'positive change experienced as a result of the struggle with a major life crisis or a traumatic event.' To some who've lost a loved one, especially if the loss is recent, it may seem obscene to suggest that any positive change could possibly be associated with that loss. The researchers clarify that they are 'not implying that traumatic events are good,' but that if, as 'most of us eventually do,' we 'face a major loss or crisis,' perhaps we 'may also experience an encounter with posttraumatic growth.'

Posttraumatic growth (PTG) is typically measured using a scale known as the Posttraumatic Growth Inventory. One of the statements in the inventory is 'I have a stronger religious faith.' A traumatic experience of loss can cause some religious believers to lose faith, but for others, the opposite may be true. Around the time my son was born, following my miscarriage, I met a mum who was welcoming a daughter following the stillbirth of her son. Losing a baby did not shake her faith. She told me she truly believed God works all things to the good. I can't fathom that perspective, though for her sake I'm glad her beliefs helped her move forward through pain. For me, goodness is not designed into any higher plan. But if we look for it, we may be able to see and find comfort in some goodness and growth that has come from loss. The Posttraumatic Growth Inventory comprises 21 statements of change that may result from crisis. Many of the statements have been true for non-religious grievers between these pages.

'New opportunities are available which would not have been otherwise' has been true for Diana and Bridget in their widowhood. Sophie would agree with 'I have a greater feeling of self-reliance' and 'I know better that I can handle difficulties,' having lost both parents at a young age.

'I have a greater sense of closeness with others,' reflects the experience of many I spoke to. When a loved one dies, some who were in our lives may cross the road and disappear, but others may come closer to us. Arthur told me that the loss of their only child, Ian, deepened his bond with his wife Wendy, if that were possible. Alison, whose daughter Lara died by suicide, spoke with gratitude of friends who remained ready to support her even after many turned-down invitations, and who were not embarrassed when she wept in public. After the death of her husband, David, step relations and exes rallied round Louisa, whom we met in chapter 11, and she realised no shared blood is required to form a strong and loving family. Sometimes bereavement brings new people into our lives, too, people whom we'd never have met, had our loved one not died. Bob formed meaningful friendships with fellow widowers at the cemetery where his dear wife Vera was buried. Alison, Kim and Alan, too, have found value in the loss communities they became part of, either in person or online.

'I have more compassion for others' resonated with Kim. She told me that before her baby died, she could be prone to judge, by the way a person looked or how they spoke, that they were not worth listening to. After losing her baby, May, Kim noticed she was more ready to listen. She realised that before she had been shutting out opportunities for connection; now, she's much more open to trying to see another person's point of view. Louisa told me that in her younger days, she would not have considered helping homeless or elderly people, but that after her husband David's death she did; she felt she had become a better person through having loved and lost him. Alan told me about the group for widows and widowers that he joined after the death of his wife, Sue. When, over time, he felt he was becoming an 'expert widower,' he was able to help new recruits ease into the group; he also passed on the benefit of his experiences at training sessions for volunteers run by bereavement charity, Cruse.

Research corroborates that those who have experienced severe adversity in their own lives, are more likely to empathise with, and spend time helping others in need. Alison, Kim and Arthur have raised money and awareness in part to keep alive the memory of the child each has lost. But they've also been motivated by a desire to help others to experience less suffering and more joy. To help others can be deeply fulfilling, creating a new sense of purpose to life after loss. I heard grief workshop leader Liese Groot-Alberts speak on a bereaved father's podcast. It was the death of her daughter, aged nearly three that propelled Groot-Alberts to work in the field of bereavement support. She described this career choice as 'a bit like turning shit into fertiliser,' an image which makes memorably vivid the growth that comes from loss, when we use our suffering to help others.

Many people find that the world looks different after the death of a loved one, and that this change in how we see things can lead to positive change in how we live our lives. Suffering and loss teach us how fragile human beings are. Until we lose a loved one, for many of us death remains largely theoretical. After experiencing loss, many people can see the value of our time here on this planet more clearly, and this heightened vision may be particularly acute for those of us who believe this is the only life we have. Many of those I spoke to would agree with items 1 and 13 on the Posttraumatic Growth Inventory: 'I changed my priorities about what is important in life' and 'I can better appreciate each day.' Louisa told me that after losing her husband David, she is no longer willing to sit in traffic jams on the North Circular. Sophie doesn't sweat the small stuff of school gate dramas, after going through the big stuff early on in life. She remembers, while others seem sometimes to forget, that what matters is to enjoy each moment with her loved ones. For Kim, all the colours of leaves and skies are more beautiful than she ever noticed them being before her baby, May, died.

None of those who told me of their losses can believe that any God or higher power works all things to the good. It can't be good that someone loved so much has gone and is never coming back. But, if we can affirm ways in which loss has changed us for the better, that's worth something.

28

THERE BUT FOR...

my story, v

When it's finally our turn, the doctor doesn't like what he sees – my little girl's glazed eyes and blue-tinged lips concern him. He lifts her top and shows how hard her tiny chest is working to pull in enough air. I hold her finger steady as he tests her oxygen saturation. The number is too low. He calls an ambulance.

The paramedic in the back with us says, 'I don't want to worry you too much, but we're going to put the lights on.' We flash along dark roads and a few times when someone doesn't move aside, the driver gives a quick burst of the siren.

Earlier, I called the safe arrival of my two children a happy ending. Of course, it was also only the beginning. My daughter has just turned one. During her first year she's had countless colds and small infections. This illness also seemed a little thing at first, but has turned more serious. At the hospital, they put prongs up her nose to deliver the extra oxygen she needs, and at frequent intervals clamp a mask over her face to give the steroid that helps open up her airways.

She's still and silent in the cot. I have the thought *she could die.* She sleeps at night and all through the next day. She's a different child from the one who said her first 'Hello' to me a couple of months earlier. She's not the girl who throws all the shoes from the shoe rack with a cheeky grin.

When she awakes she is lethargic, has no interest in her milk. The nurses are monitoring her hydration and becoming worried, saying they'll have to get an IV line in. She has been screaming and struggling when it's mask time. I don't want them to stick a cannula in her as well. I coax and try repeatedly and eventually get her to drink a little from her bottle.

By the fourth day, she seems to be heading in the right direction. They say we'll see if we can make it through the night without the oxygen. We try but her levels slip again and she has to have the prongs back in. On the fifth night, she does it - breathes unaided - and on the morning of the sixth day she's allowed for the first time to the hospital playroom. We have reached the far side of the crisis.

What I remember most from that time is her face, the roundness gone from her cheeks, the colour gone from her skin. We were supposed to have been in Bulgaria; it would have been her first meeting with her grandparents there, her Baba and Dyado. Instead, they see her on screen. Baba's reaction, as translated by Niko is, 'There's nothing left of her but two big eyes!'

It takes some time for my little girl to regain the lost weight, the lost strength. But a few months later, we make it to Bulgaria. Baba opens the door, grabs her grandchild from me, holds her close.

'There but for the grace of God go I.' The expression is part of my cultural background and sometimes springs to mind. I have my children. I have my husband. I still have my parents. I am alive and very grateful. But, when 'There but for...' springs to my mind, I reject it. I don't believe in any God who through His grace is choosing to protect me and the ones I love from harm. I don't believe I'm any more special than those who've lost their closest loved ones, or who face the possibly imminent loss of their own life. I've just been mostly lucky so far.

You and I drew different tickets in the lottery of life. The time and place we're born, who we're born to, the genetic mix and the nurture we receive and a million other factors we can't control or fathom, determine how our lives play out. But it's my belief, in one way our situation is the same: we're all equally unloved by any God. I find a human solidarity in that. We hold each other close while we still can.

I remember to be grateful for my winning ticket when I think of people I've known, my age, who died when we were in our teens and twenties. On a

144

day soon after I started secondary school, I was chatting to a classmate, Rosie, and asked about her siblings. She told me she had a younger sister and then said something like 'I also had a sister who would have been 14.' I didn't understand the grammar – it took me a while to grasp she was calmly telling me her older sister died. That was almost incomprehensible to me. Rosie's sister died due to cystic fibrosis. Rosie had the condition, too. I admired how she didn't let CF stop her living to the full and having fun. The summer we finished our GCSEs, she, I and a bunch of other girls went on a seaside holiday together. Rosie died soon after we left school, aged 19. Though the two of us weren't really close, for many years I saw her in my dreams. Thoughts of her made me decide I wanted to include the story of someone with cystic fibrosis in this book.

Most of us assume we'll live to see old age. I wanted to understand what it's like to know from early on that time for you is likely to be shorter than for the average person. How does that knowledge shape a life? Tristan shared his story with me.

29

TRISTAN

how to live knowing time's not endless

Last October, Tristan lost all interest in the things he usually enjoyed. People close to him had struggled with depression and anxiety, so he recognised the symptoms, but it was the first time that Tristan hadn't felt like Tristan. It was frightening. He felt a flatness, a sense that he could sleep for weeks, and he didn't know where these feelings came from and whether they would leave again. Or, *is this my life now?*

Tristan is 24 years old and has cystic fibrosis. CF is a genetic condition that causes sticky mucus to build up in the lungs and digestive system. Over time, organs become increasingly damaged and - though treatments are improving and life expectancy is increasing – CF remains a life-shortening condition. Tristan has a memory from when he was around seven or eight. He'd just got out of the bath and his mum was towelling him dry and helping him into his pyjamas and he said 'I don't want to die. If we die, we're not here any more.' Probably he is assigning too much significance to this memory in retrospect. He isn't sure what put the thought of death into his mind. He knows it wasn't connected to any news he'd had at the CF clinic. It will have been something he'd read or seen on TV that had scared him a bit. And he was at that age of beginning to understand that death's a thing, that life isn't a given forever. There was some dawning awareness that *all this* is temporary, including this moment in a bathroom between a mother and her child. His mum said something like 'Of course you're not

146

going to' and really, she was right, he wasn't going to any time soon, he wasn't ill.

When he was first diagnosed as a baby, the doctor who delivered the news sent his parents away with a gloomy picture of how things would be. They thought they were taking home a really sick child, who would not be able to interact with other kids in the playground, who would have to stay inside for fear of catching bugs, but they quickly realised Tristan could have a normal childhood. Though it may sound odd to talk of luck when you've been born with a life-limiting genetic illness, Tristan has been lucky. Lucky to have been born in an area that was trialling the heel prick test, so that he was diagnosed as a newborn and treatment could start straight away; lucky, perhaps – though he's no expert on this – that he has only one copy of the particular mutation delta F508 and not two; and lucky perhaps most of all in his parents, who brought him up to think of his CF not as a burden but simply part of his normal routine. He knew that life for him involved little grains sprinkled on his yoghurt (of Creon, to help him digest food), physiotherapy each morning and evening, (to loosen the mucus in his lungs) and occasional visits to the clinic.

Tristan was 11 when he was first admitted to hospital. People with CF are prone to picking up bacterial infections, for which they need intravenous antibiotics, typically requiring a two-week hospital stay. The first time Tristan needed to go in, he was very nervous. When they were about to put the line in, he tried to get off the bed because he wanted to run somewhere very far away. But they gave him Entonox, so that it wouldn't hurt, and he started feeling floaty and tingly in quite a pleasant way! Each day he was in hospital, his parents gave him a little present, so that each night he had something to look forward to in the morning: a Simpsons book, pyjamas (which he still wears 13 years later) and a 1GB memory stick, which seemed like a world of data at the time! Both his grandmothers wrote to him frequently, letting him know what they were up to, and even though what they were up to was sometimes quite banal, it was nice to feel he was still connected to people out there who cared about him, who were going through this experience with him. And now that both of his grandmothers have died, it is good to have these cards and letters with their handwriting preserved, these marks that could only have been made by one hand out of seven billion, that were made by that hand on that day with that pen. It makes him smile to see the sexy nurse joke on the front of the card his cheeky Grandma Cherry sent to 11-year-old him.

People sometimes express to Tristan something like 'Having CF must be so difficult for you.' But it is not as if something was taken away from him: life with CF is all he's ever known. Of course, two-week hospital stays are no one's idea of fun. Around day nine is usually when Tristan starts feeling shit about the situation, sick of the rubbish food and of staring at the same walls. CF sufferers need to be kept separate from each other, due to the risk of cross-infection with harmful bugs; having your own hospital room is a blessing in some ways, but it's lonely. What helped most growing up was that one of Tristan's parents would always be with him in that hospital room. Now, as an adult, if he's upset, he's able to better articulate what's wrong; when he was younger there'd be tears more often. Tristan's mum is a very emotional person herself, so if he cried, she'd cry, but they'd have a sort of huggle to get through it.

Growing up, Tristan was never able to meet other children with CF. So for him, CF was just what *he* had to do in *his* life, as opposed to something that happened in the wider world. Then one day, walking home, some friends from secondary school came up to him: 'Tristan, are you going to die?' It was a bit of a shock. Tristan knew that life expectancy with CF was lower, in the somethings - some figure that felt unconnected to *his* life. He told his friends, 'No, I'm not planning to.' He was able to reassure them they'd been taught outdated information, that treatments had improved for people with CF. Life expectancy and lung transplants weren't really subjects that came up at home or clinic visits: he knew about CF as it related to him, and generally he was fine.

While many parents are able to step back a little during the teen years, Tristan's parents still needed to protect his health. They'd remind him to take his tablets and sit next to him on the sofa while he breathed into his PEP mask, ensuring his breaths out were reaching the pressure needed to keep his airways clear. When the time came for Tristan to go off to uni he was apprehensive about how it would feel to be far from his parents and alone. He wasn't one for clubbing – he didn't like the idea of getting drunk and losing control, and knew his liver was at increased risk of damage due to CF. He knew there would be times when his flatmates would go out at night and he'd be on his own. It turned out he quite liked this. The student accommodation looked over a cityscape defined by coloured lights and was next to a busy roundabout. There was something weirdly comforting about seeing cars drive past at night, even about hearing police and ambulance sirens, while he was lying in bed trying to get to sleep. Some people would be thinking *something's going off, there's trouble,* but to Tristan it was *yeah, there's trouble, there's always trouble everywhere, but someone is on their way to sort it out.* Though in some ways he wasn't a typical student – his only experience of alcohol was a sip of someone's Sex on the Beach once – he did share with the others living away from home for the first time that excitement, that high of realising he was creating his own world now. And he found love.

Tristan and Ruby were friends for the first year, before it became something more. She knew he had CF, but didn't know much about what that meant and Tristan wanted to be honest: CF means physio every morning, every evening, no exceptions; it means hospital stays from time to time; it means trouble having children, probably the need to go through IVF, because 98% of men with CF are infertile; and it means not knowing what the future holds, what the trajectory of the disease will look like. Life might not be an easy ride – and he wasn't trying to make it any easier either: three months into their relationship, Tristan ran the London marathon. The strain on his body meant two weeks in hospital and then, because he still hadn't quite recovered, he needed another hospital stay two months later. In their first six months together, Tristan was in hospital for four weeks. Ruby's mum asked her 'Are you sure you want to keep going through this? You do have a choice – are you sure this is the life you want?' Ruby said, 'Yeah, it's horrible, but I don't want not to be with him, I don't want to be with someone else so I can have an easier life.' Tristan learnt of this conversation later, but at the time, Ruby's commitment to him was already very clear. Being ill in hospital makes you emotionally vulnerable, you feel like you're a burden, but Ruby assured him he was not. She went to stay at his parents' house for a week because that was close to the hospital he'd been admitted to. Staying with your boyfriend's parents when your boyfriend isn't there and you're only a few months into the relationship – it's quite a big deal, but Ruby didn't make it seem so. Going through these periods of illness as a team, intensified, accelerated their relationship.

Tristan felt immensely lucky to have such support from his family and from Ruby. He was aware there was a whole world of CF to be found online, but he never felt the urge to seek out fellow CF sufferers. He sort of felt there wasn't much point, because the risk of cross-infection meant it wouldn't be a good idea to meet someone else with CF in person. Also, because CF's a different journey for everyone, Tristan was wary about how it might feel to connect with someone more ill than him, or, even, should he become more ill down the line, how it might feel to be connected to someone with CF who was still well. But then one evening in his second year at uni, he was considering how many chips to bake in the oven for dinner. He had to be careful because he knew eating too many would trigger his digestive problems. One of his flatmates told him to 'Man up and eat the chips,' and though they meant no harm, and it was just a little thing, it reminded Tristan no one around him could really *get it*, even those closest to him, because they didn't *have it*. So he started looking at Instagram and Facebook and he reached out. Gradually, he formed more and more online links to others with CF and that has felt good. There have been times when someone else with CF has spoken about their feelings and experiences and he's had that moment: *ah! That's exactly the same for me.* There's something nice in that sense of recognition. Of course, you need to have more than a genetic condition in common to develop a true friendship; there are a few people now, with whom he shares more than that one thing, whom he counts as real friends.

As he became more involved in the online world of CF, Tristan formed an idea for a project that would raise awareness about the condition amongst the general public, while also providing the reassurance of a realistic picture to the parents of newly-diagnosed children. He wanted to help bewildered parents who have no idea about CF, who are likely to look online and find awful things about kids dying young. Through his project, Tristan presents the stories of CF that are really good, alongside those that are really bad, but also the stories of people with CF just living normal lives. Though he's self-conscious about how this might sound, Tristan has always wanted to make an impact. It means quite a lot to him, the idea that his being here, his being born and dying, could actually change the world in some way. His CF project is one of the things that gives him a sense of purpose; he hopes he's helping people to be better informed and less afraid.

As Tristan began to speak to more and more people about their experiences with CF, he was surprised to realise that many CF sufferers have a different perspective on their illness from his own. Those based in the US, where Christian beliefs are still much more of a cultural norm, often speak of finding comfort in a belief that God has a plan for them, that the difficulties they face because of CF have been designed by God to test them and help them grow. Religion never figured much in Tristan's childhood, though his mother's beliefs are loosely Christian. His parents didn't have him or his brother christened, because they thought it was a decision a person should make themselves. There were hymns and prayers at primary school, but as he learnt and thought more, Tristan concluded what many others had before him: that whole all-loving, all-knowing, all-powerful triangle doesn't make sense. Tristan's not for looking down on people who have different beliefs from his own. It does confuse him, though, if people believe they've been given this illness by a God who loves them, why was that, how does that happen? He's not about to argue anyone out of what gives them comfort, though. People living with very difficult situations try to get through however they can.

As Tristan became more immersed in his CF project, he was speaking to people in very serious situations, including someone whose health was deteriorating while on the waiting list for a double lung transplant, and someone else who later died from complications following a transplant operation. Hearing people's experiences affected Tristan because he got to know these people, he began to care about them; he was also becoming more aware of the paths disease progression can take with CF, in a way that suddenly felt threatening to him. He'd known previously about the many problems that can come with CF, such as diabetes and antibiotic resistance. Now though, it all felt much more real. Tristan's not someone who does things by half – he tends to get consumed by projects that he's working on. CF went from something he spent a short time on each day – when taking tablets or doing physio – to something he was thinking of from first thing in the morning to last thing at night. He had scheduled work on the project to be completed weekly and for a while he was on track. When he began to feel a sense of weight descend, when the project became a chore and no longer excited him, at first Tristan ploughed on. But it got to the point that he knew he should speak to somebody.

Studies have shown that people with CF are more likely to experience depression and anxiety than the general population. Because of this vulnerability and the fact untreated mental health problems can lead to a deterioration in physical health too, people with CF have access to a therapist when needed. Tristan's very grateful for this, especially given the current underfunding of mental health services. Tristan's therapist understood he didn't want to let people down, but she pointed out he'd been working so hard trying to help others he'd forgotten to look after himself. She told him 'You've got a free pass because you're not well. You don't have to work now – everyone will understand. You need time just to relax and recover.' It was good to hear this from a professional.

So Tristan put his life on hold. His parents came down and drove him and his fiancé back to his childhood home. In the car, Tristan's legs began to jerk erratically, he started shaking violently all over. It was alarming because he'd never experienced anything like that before, but Ruby recognised he was having a panic attack. She was familiar with grounding techniques, intended to bring you back to the present moment. She was saying to Tristan, 'Your feet are on the floor, you're firmly in your seat' to help him see the safety of his situation. When they got home, his mum gave him a hug and let him know although these feelings were new to him, everything he was going through was totally normal. She knew this from personal experience, as well as her experiences as a nurse. She reassured him there was nothing wrong with him *per se*, he was just going through a tough time. Then Tristan lay on the sofa with Ruby, under a blanket because the weather was getting cold, and he immediately felt relaxed. He was at home with Ruby and his parents for about two weeks – being looked after, going on gentle walks, watching Pointless every day at 5 o'clock, with the pleasing sense each day he was a little further forward in getting back to being himself.

Since then, Tristan is more aware of when he needs to take a break. If he starts to feel a bit strange, he'll talk to Ruby, maybe his mum, and he's able to identify a bit more why he might be feeling certain things. At the beginning of this year he started mindfulness meditation, using the app Headspace. It helps to have ten minutes in the day when he focuses only on his breath and nothing else matters. Running can be meditative as well, when you forget what you're doing and fall into a natural rhythm of one foot after the other. Exercise has been ingrained in him as a key part of maintaining physical health, but lately he's come to appreciate its benefits for his mental health, too. If he goes for a run first thing, the day's already got this energy to it that makes him feel he cannot fail. Gaining an understanding of mindfulness meditation, and conversations with his therapist, have helped him better handle negative thoughts. It's no use trying to stop yourself from having them. If someone tells you not to think about a white bear, it's all you think of. But if you let the thoughts come and go and don't buy into them too much, don't let them define you, you start to feel ok. So he reminds himself what part of the journey he's on with CF. All any of us have is now – the past is gone and the future isn't here yet. He can't know what will happen down the line, but right now Tristan's doing well.

His mum has said she wishes she could take CF away for him, but he's actually not sure he'd want her to. There's a lot of horrible things that come with CF, but also lots of ways it's shaped his life positively. He knows that many people with CF feel the same – that they are who they are because of CF and taking it away wouldn't necessarily be a wonderful thing. As much as CF can limit a person's life, it can also be a motivation to push through limits. He's scared of not doing things while he still can. It can be difficult sometimes to have that fear there in the background. But he channels it in positive ways. Not many guys these days want to pop the question at 22, but Tristan did. He was pretty sure from early on that Ruby was the person he wanted to share life with, and luckily she felt the same! None of us know how long we've got and that's even more the case with CF. Tristan wants children with Ruby, he wants grandchildren and he wants as long as he can have in the company of his loved ones.

Tristan doesn't believe that any God gave him CF to challenge him or help him grow, but he does believe that having this condition has spurred him on to challenge *himself*. Stand-up comedy is one of Tristan's hobbies. Whether he's good or bad at it is not for him to say, but it buoys him up to think there are people out there who'd like to try, but can't bring themselves to do it. Just by getting up on stage he has achieved something. He's pretty sure, too, he wouldn't have run the London marathon if he didn't have CF. He built his running up from nothing, with the 'Couch to 5K' programme. It took a huge effort for him to get to that point, to be able to run 5k non-stop. From there, he did a 10k, then a half marathon, and started thinking *I'd love to run the marathon. Why don't I try? I'm not there yet, but I can get there.* Because CF's a progressive illness, there was no guarantee he'd be at the same level health-wise one year on. He put in for the ballot and got a place first time. He decided to raise money for the Cystic Fibrosis Trust. Someone from a local news programme came round and asked why he wanted to run the marathon; Tristan said he was running on behalf of all of those who cannot run themselves. They spoke to his mum too, asked her 'Are you nervous?' She said, 'It's done, he'll do it.' Tristan was running for 6 hours and 40 minutes and that was a long old slog, but whenever he was struggling, he'd listen to that bit of audio through his headphones - of his Mum saying: 'Anything he puts his mind to, he'll do it, no matter how long it takes.' And he did. He lost a worrying amount of weight; it took two hospital stays to coax the pounds back on. These days he mostly sticks to 5ks. Ruby and his parents would be horrified if he floated the idea of running a marathon again; probably he won't. But he's glad he ran one. When he crossed the finish line, he was conscious of not wanting just to let that moment go by: he breathed it in.

30

BEFORE I DIE

and the death awareness movement

Tristan has never had that luxury many young people enjoy, to live as if he is immortal. He's always understood he isn't physically indestructible. He needs to take care with diet and exercise and doesn't drink alcohol. But in a way, those living with a delusion of immortality are the less lucky ones. Tristan's understanding that his time's not endless isn't something he would wish to change.

Most people try to look at death as little as possible for as long as possible, and in the 21st century in the West, that can often be quite a long time. In 1841, the average newborn girl in the UK was not expected to see her 43rd birthday, while the average baby boy was not expected to reach his 41st. Cleaner living conditions, vaccinations and developments in medical technology have contributed to dramatic increases in life expectancy, with the latest UK figures putting life expectancy at birth for males at 79.3 years, and for females at 82.9 years. Most of us will live into old age, and can, for a number of decades, push down thoughts of death as something too distant to pose us any real threat. Yet, in recent years, a growing 'death awareness' movement is spreading the word that being willing to look at death and talk about it can help us to more fully *live*.

In 2011, influenced by the ideas of sociologist Bernard Crettaz, Jon Underwood held the first 'Death Café' at his home in Hackney, East

London. Since then, thousands of Death Cafés have been held in 73 countries around the world. At a Death Café, people gather to eat cake, drink tea and discuss death. A Death Café convenes with no appointed leader, nor agenda, meaning that people are free to speak of whatever is on their mind in relation to death. The aim is 'to increase awareness of death with a view to helping people make the most of their (finite) lives'.

Candy Chang's 'Before I Die' project has a similar aim. After losing a loved one, the artist found contemplating death brought a sense of clarity and gratitude to her life, but that she 'struggled to maintain this perspective.' She observed that 'it's easy to get caught up in the day-to-day and forget what really matters to you,' and also noticed 'how much we avoid talking about death.' Chang created the first Before I Die wall on the side of an abandoned house in New Orleans. She painted the wall with black chalkboard paint, and then repeatedly stencilled, in white, the prompt 'Before I die I want to _____.' By the next day, the wall was entirely filled, with sentiments including 'see my daughter graduate,' 'follow my childhood dream' and 'see the leaves change many times.' Since then, over 5000 Before I Die walls have been created, helping many people around the world to remember that our time on this earth is finite and precious.

Brian, a London-based humanist funeral celebrant, told me about the time he, with a group of others, brought a Before I Die wall to his local area. Brian knows many would prefer not face the reality that we all die. As a consequence, when a loved one dies, family and friends are often left with regrets about what remained unsaid or undone. The idea was for the wall to start a conversation in the community about what matters in this life. At the planning meeting, Brian's friend Christine turned up to get involved. She let those gathered know that, as she had recently been given a terminal diagnosis, the question of what she would like to do before she died had become particularly pertinent for her. She struggled to think of how she might encapsulate her response in a few chalk words, though. She went away and wrote a longer piece, which, the following year, Brian read out at her memorial service. In it, Christine notes that many people desire to see more of the world before leaving it, but that she would rather be in the company of family and best friends than on a cruise liner squashed in with new people. Over spectacular scenery, she would choose weeding her own garden and warm hugs with her grandchildren. She summarises that she doesn't want anything to change in her life; she is happy doing what she is doing, being where she is, and with the people she is with. She concludes that, in fact, she can answer the question posed by the blackboard in one word: what more does she want to see or do before she dies? Nothing.

What an inspiringly affirmative 'nothing.' When we live with an awareness that our time is limited, we can choose to focus on those things that matter to us most, so that we reach the end of life unburdened by regrets. Tristan's awareness that cystic fibrosis may shorten his life spurs him to seize his dreams right now: to face his fears and perform stand-up comedy, run a marathon, and propose to the woman he loves. That an awareness of our own mortality can help us to truly live is an inspiring thought – but for Tristan, and for me, it isn't the whole story.

31

FLIPPING THE STORY

the days on which we live

Charlie Brown: Some day, we will all die, Snoopy!
Snoopy: True, but on all the other days, we will not.

Charles M. Schulz, *Peanuts*

I said in the previous chapter that most people try to look at death as little as possible for as long as possible. If that is true, then I am not most people. Death has always loomed too large for me to ignore. It is possible to be *too* aware of death. Most of us live for many thousands of days - we only die on one of those days. Snoopy is a wise dog and I am training myself to think more like him.

Our brains have a negativity bias. As positive psychologist Miriam Akhtar explains, we are evolutionarily 'wired to notice what's wrong before we notice what's right, a part of the safety mechanism that kicks in whenever we're under threat. So we're aware of the runaway car headed our way and are not distracted by appreciating the beautiful view.' Though this evolved trait may be useful at times, it's much less useful for us than it would have been for our ancestors on the savannah and this habit of looking for the negatives can be detrimental to our mental health.

Isn't it sad we're all going to die? has been one of the core thoughts of my first decades of life. But it is not the only way to tell our human story. Secular thinker Dale McGowan points out that, though 'we tend to think of life as our natural condition and death as some sort of affront to that condition,' in truth that presumption should be flipped on its head: 'since the stuff that makes you up has always been here and will always be here, nonexistence can be seen as our normal condition. But for one short blip in that vast nonexistence, pop – here you are. Existing. Conscious. Instead of seeing death as an outrage, this view allows us to see death as the universal norm and *life* as the giddy exception.' These days I try more often to choose the thought *aren't we lucky we get to live?*

Each of us is here at extremely long odds. A particular sperm had to penetrate a particular egg and all conditions had to be right for the pregnancy to thrive. When we look back further, at all the moments necessary to our moment of conception – the happenstance circumstances through which each pair of our ancestors created each particular life that led to ours – we may begin to appreciate the extent of our good fortune in coming into being. Despite the mind-bogglingly long odds of it being so, here we are.

If Iain had lived, I wouldn't be here. My parents had two girls and felt their family was not yet complete. 18 weeks into her third pregnancy, Mum began bleeding heavily. The doctor came and couldn't understand why, already having two, she should be so upset. In hospital, after the procedure to make sure everything was cleared away, they said they could tell her the sex if she would like. She said no – she didn't want to imagine the possibility of a particular child. Later, she couldn't help but do so. He would have been a boy, and she'd have called him Iain, with two 'i's.

After a few years, a third girl joined the family. Dad had worried a third might feel left out - I was conceived to be her playmate. Mum speaks of the pregnancy she lost, with a hint of wistfulness she never had a boy, which she keeps entirely separate from her fierce love for each of her four girls. She doesn't make the direct link I do – if she'd had Iain she'd never have had me. This is just one of many ways I might never have existed. Six months pregnant with me, my mum started to bleed. She was frightened. This looked like the beginning of another loss. The doctor told her to go home and rest. She had to move as little as possible for the next three months, parenting three children from the settee. She managed to hold onto me. When the day came for my arrival, we seemed to be on the final strait, all systems go, until the midwife shouted 'Stop, don't push!' I was stuck. They injected Mum with something that knocked her instantly out.

When she woke they told her that off in another room somewhere, born by emergency caesarean, she had a baby girl.

I am here and happy to be so and try to remember to focus on that. An 'attitude of gratitude' is linked to better mental health. Of specific relevance for this book, gratitude has been linked both to lower levels of death anxiety amongst older adults, and to higher levels of subjective well-being in people living with a terminal illness. Consciously cultivating positive emotions is a way to combat the brain's negativity bias. The expression of gratitude has traditionally been associated with religious practice. The faithful may offer up thanks to their God(s) for bounty received, for being kept safe from harm, for life itself. One of my non-religious interviewees, a woman in her eighties, was puzzled when I asked her about gratitude. To whom or what should she be grateful? Most I spoke to did feel and express gratitude, not *to* any divine entity, but *for* all that is good in life. Studies show the active practice of gratitude improves well-being. Writing lists or journals expressing gratitude; regularly thinking about what we're grateful for; and visiting someone to whom we're grateful, to express our gratitude in person, have all been demonstrated as effective ways to boost well-being. We can train our brains to notice the good more than the bad.

Tristan hopes to live a long life, but sometimes the knowledge that many people with cystic fibrosis don't, weighs heavy. He told me how, debilitated by fears of future possibilities, he gradually found his way back to enjoying life through self-care, regular exercise, and taking ten minutes each day when he focuses on his breath and nothing else matters. Mindfulness meditation, which derives from a spiritual practice in Buddhism, has been adopted by many as a secular practice that can help maintain good mental health. Tristan has made meditation a part of his daily routine, because it helps him to bring his attention back to life in the present moment.

Tristan and I both have a vulnerability to bouts of anxiety and low mood. For me, as for Tristan, running and other forms of exercise often help. I've dabbled in meditation. The habit hasn't stuck yet – maybe some day. But I think I'm getting better at challenging negative thought patterns and looking for the other side of the story. Grateful thoughts come more easily to me now than they did before I began the reading and the conversations of this book. Death looms less large, when I look with gratitude at the days I've had, the one I'm living in and those likely still ahead. In this, Paul, whom you'll meet next, has been one of my teachers.

32

PAUL AND JENNY

life is one big learning curve

Paul is heading into extra time, another summer; last summer he was told he had around a year to live. Besides which, at 82 years old he has already outstripped the life expectancy for males in the UK. Paul considers himself a lucky man.

He has advanced cancer of the oesophagus. Back in February, following ten sessions of radiotherapy at quite a high level, Paul's difficulty swallowing became such that he was unable to take in any food or liquids; he landed up in hospital with a nasal tube sustaining him. After a week of this, when the situation was looking irreversible, a nurse came wanting to show Paul how to manage his own tube feeding at home with a portable pack. He thought then about a letter he'd once read, written by a Russian soldier who'd been captured in the Battle of Stalingrad. This soldier knew it was the intention of his German captors to shoot him dead along with his comrades the next morning. The letter contains no hope or expectation of the outcome being otherwise; instead he writes 'Why can't they get it over with?' Paul wasn't quite at the point of asking that himself, but he was not far from it. *Because what is the point of being kept alive if the quality of life is gone?* Paul told the nurse this portable pack was not for him, that when he managed to escape from hospital, he would enjoy his usual portion of the finest fish and chips in his local town. To prove his intent, he tried a cup of tea, and when that went down ok, asked for another one. The next day he managed a light breakfast, then a light lunch and said 'I think you can take these tubes out now,' which they did, and the following day he was allowed home.

So now it is July, and Paul still hasn't come to the point of asking that Russian soldier's question. Swallowing continues to be challenging, especially in the morning, when he has many pills to get down; he manages with tea and water. His appetite has diminished, so he makes supplemental drinks, to keep his calories and nutrients topped up. On a good day, though, he can manage tomatoes on toast for breakfast. Later there might be some naughty treat – pork belly, lemon tart with passion fruit, perhaps a glass or two of wine. It is a delight to be able to enjoy these things, still.

On a typical day, after breakfast, his lady friend Beatrice, who lives in the flat across the landing, will come over and they'll walk to the local shop together, buy the papers and a few bits. They'll spend time on the crossword, then one of them will prepare lunch. Around two, Paul will feel very noddy and he'll sleep for a couple of hours. Later, he and Beatrice will meet again, have tea and spend the evening perhaps reading or watching television. Any bits of the crossword that caused bother earlier, they'll think about and try to solve together before retiring for the night. On Monday afternoons, they play cards with a couple of others who live in the block, using Victorian coins to bet, and that's a bit of fun. There are things – for now there are enough things – that make Paul's day-to-day life enjoyable. At the same time, it is not a horrible or terrifying thought that this life will soon come to an end.

Paul does not believe there'll be another life after the one he's living now. He's a scientist, with a love for the natural world; when he reads about and looks around at the world we have, he does think *something has happened here that's rather marvellous, there must be something that sort of caused this thing to happen.* After school, he trained as an analytical chemist and was amazed at the activities of single-celled organisms under the microscope. Later, as a researcher in the food technology industry, he was astounded at the variety of flavours and fragrances that come from plants. To Paul, it seems so pompous, amidst these natural phenomena, for humans to think there's some supreme entity looking after only us. Paul believes we all just take our chances: bacteria, human or whatever.

He is at ease with his belief that there's no heaven. He's worked in lots of different places for lots of different people; often during his career, the thought crossed Paul's mind *if there's a heaven and you're there, I won't be very happy!* Up till he was around 70 years old, there was something bothersome for Paul in the thought that one day he would not exist, but now – and he can't really say why or how this change has taken place – to contemplate that fact is bothersome no longer. Perhaps it is because, by 70, Paul had done a fair amount of living to look back on. He'd worked in many countries, learnt a little of many languages and cultures. Near the border of Zambia with Angola he had an AK47 poked at his throat by a guard who suspected him of transporting something less innocuous than pineapples – and he lived to tell this tale and others for several decades more.

This is Paul's fourth cancer. The first, in his prostate, was diagnosed around five years ago. That diagnosis was a shock because until then he'd been pretty healthy and active, he hadn't needed to deal with hospitals or doctors other than for the odd thing. The local Macmillan centre was wonderful though – they cured the prostate cancer for him. And then they cured his bladder cancer and skin cancer too. When you get cancer for the fourth time, you don't feel devastated, you think *oh well, more of the same thing.* Then the oncologist explained how extensive this cancer was, that an operation would not be possible. Chemo and radiotherapy were options offering the possibility of a little more time. Paul tried both – the chemo had no impact, but it seems the radio had some because he's still standing and doesn't feel on his last legs quite yet.

Beatrice keeps him motivated. When he's had a bad spell, being sick and lying in bed for days, she's the one who'll bring him out of it: 'Come on, you've got to get up for a few hours.' He has a rowing machine in his flat and before the cancers, he used to row for about a quarter of an hour each day; with the prostate cancer his backside was too sore for that, and now if he were to get down on that machine, he'd have a job to get back up! He realises, though, that exercise is important whatever stage of life you're at. The walk with Beatrice to the shops and back is just over a mile, and that's still something. Paul wasn't looking for a relationship when Beatrice came knocking. He'd been married twice, divorced twice – 54 married years in total – and he sort of felt he'd done his bit! There's a community organisation that's very helpful in taking residents who are interested out on day trips; Beatrice asked the manager of the block of flats whether she knew of anyone who might go with her, and she said 'Why don't you ask Paul – he lives just opposite.' Beatrice did ask. Paul hesitated, then replied, 'Why don't you go with Pam next door?' Somehow, though, they got together. And it's good. They talk openly, keep each other company, she makes great cakes when his son and daughter visit.

That Simon and Jenny *do* visit once a month, and that they text and phone, is a source of happiness for Paul, because his relationships with his children haven't always been easy. At the age of 70, he retired from work and left their mother. He'd met someone he loved and made a decision to live a little more while he still could. He'd been working in Romania, when they were just about to join the EU, training people in hygiene standards for food products. Maria was his interpreter, 29 years old. Paul was sanguine about the whole thing, saying 'Oh, she won't stay with me for ever – probably five years or something,' but they got married and were happy for a time.

Not everyone was happy of course. Jenny helped her mother take her dad's stuff to the tip. Part of her felt uneasy doing it, but her mum said 'He's not coming back for his old shoes, is he?' It was like chucking out her dad. There was a kind of pre-grieving then; though she was 44, she still felt on some level as though her dad had left *her*. When she saw her dad, which wasn't often, he and Maria would sort of whisper into each other, and it was as if Maria was the spokesperson for the couple. She was now the one who'd buy Christmas or birthday presents from the two of them for Jenny. One time, Maria had knitted Jenny a poncho and a hat. When presented with them, Jenny put them on, but afterwards she chucked them in the bin. There were some awkward family lunches hosted by Maria, at which Simon's kids – Paul's grandkids – would sit in total silence. Jenny remembers one time Maria took her aside and said, 'You and your brother never call,' and Jenny answered, 'We don't care.' The confusing thing was, Maria was very nice, and she and Paul did have a nice relationship. But when her dad hugged her, she didn't really hug him back, because on some chemical, gut level, she hated him. Towards the end of Paul and Maria's relationship, Jenny met them at a restaurant; Maria arrived with a huge lock she'd just bought, for the motorbike she would zip around on while Paul used his free bus pass. All told, the marriage lasted eight years. Paul took its ending well; Maria's new partner seemed pleasant the afternoon they met and wandered round a gallery together.

He was embarking on something new, himself, having been diagnosed with prostate cancer. Paul's life has been made up of many different chapters: something new comes up, you learn what it's all about, then you get on and do whatever must be done. What they don't tell you in school is that life is just one great big learning curve from start to finish. Of course, there are some things you'd rather not learn, but there's usually something engaging, something of interest in the process. At the same time Paul was diagnosed with prostate cancer, Jenny's partner Alex received the same news. So they've been through it together – the disease, its treatments and its repercussions. A sympathy developed between the three of them. It was a leveller – as if there were no more old and young, man and woman, father and daughter – just people all getting older and having to face the problems that age brings. They were able to talk candidly about male members and bowel movements, and the candour spread to other aspects of their lives. When, for the first time, Jenny confronted her dad about his relationship with Maria – 'Didn't you ever think it was weird you had a wife 15 years younger than your own daughter?' – he replied, 'Well, your mum's last affair got a bit serious…' Her mum's infidelity was news to Jenny, but later confirmed by others. As time goes on, she realises she doesn't blame either parent for what happened. Her mum was left alone in the village much of the time; her dad was off working abroad, meeting new people all the time, living a different kind of life.

Alex's prostate cancer was aggressive and advanced, a horrible shock. But he got through it and it kicked Jenny into a proposal. They'd been together since she was 19. After 32 years together, they got married. Jenny didn't invite her dad; her mum had felt the ending of the marriage as a bereavement and couldn't be in the same space as Paul. Of course, Paul would have liked to have been there, but he was glad to have the chance, ahead of the day, to check out the venue with Jenny and Alex. The woman took them through the service, went through what would happen when, and then they had a meal. Jenny said to her dad, 'Effectively, you've done it now,' and he took that alright: 'Well, I can see photos of my daughter's wedding, can't I?'

After his relationship with Maria ended, facing the fact he was now alone and unwell, Paul organised himself a place in sheltered accommodation, so he could remain as independent as possible, but know support was in place should he require it. He's always thought of himself as solo, in a way. Paul was a boy in World War II. His father died when he was three, and his mother was a Wren, so Paul was sent to Monmouth to be looked after by his grandparents. He was a spectacle-wearing, boss-eyed kid who knew no one; the other kids pushed him away. That may be why Paul formed the belief that in life we go our own way. That may have been why, with his third cancer, he didn't even bother telling his kids for quite a while. A steady pattern of communication and support has emerged, though. Jenny's life is at the other end of the country, but once a month, she and her brother Simon come and spend the day with Paul. It feels like getting back to being a family; they talk and laugh and get on. Paul always tries to think of something to show them that will be of interest. He's never been one of those who shut down and withdraw from a world that is changing rapidly around them. He's good with technology, so he can stream a bit of a documentary online, or show them that the converted monastery in France, where they lived for six months as a family when the kids were small, is now an Airbnb they might want to revisit some time.

164

So, now it is September, and more than a year since Paul was told he had around a year to live. Things have moved along a little for Paul, with the season, not for the better, of course. The cancer has spread to his liver now, so there's not much more medically to be done, apart from keeping him as comfortable as possible. It's really just a question of time, and Paul doesn't particularly want that time to fly. When the kids visit, the focus now is on clearing the bookshelves in his bedroom, to make space for a hospital bed, if that is needed. It's been an enjoyable experience, for the three of them to go through all the books and DVDs, chatting about Paul's wide-ranging interests and experiences, from languages, to science, food technology and art. He shows them the slide rule with which he used to make calculations as a young man. He tells them to have fun, because it's soon all over. They get it officially recorded that, should he suffer a cardiac arrest, he doesn't want resuscitation to be attempted. They discuss his wishes for a low-fuss, low-cost direct cremation, and then for his ashes to be scattered on the Suffolk coast. But when Jenny notices that even after clearing out his books, her dad's still getting packages from Amazon, he tells her, 'Well, I'm still interested in life!'

There are so many strands to a life; to an extent you can choose what narrative you weave from them. You can say this happened and that happened and it was terrible or you can say *this* happened and *that* happened and it was wonderful! Paul tries to be positive, and hopeful that at the end things won't be too bad. He's never thought of himself as anyone particularly special, but he did try to help people with his work, which involved coming up with solutions for problems: devising solar drying panels for apple rings, or advising on packaging that would reduce food spoilage. So you sort of hope some good has come from your life.

These days, Paul spends a lot of time sitting in his armchair. To be so languid and listless is a strange feeling for a man who used to hop on and off a plane a hundred times a year. But there are compensations. He takes more from nature than he ever could when he was young and rushing round, he takes it all in now. He enjoys the changes in the light throughout the day, the sense of movement you can get - though all is still - just through sunlight. He feels privileged to see the seasons changing. In July, he saw the buddleias blossom and butterflies bustle round. It's amazing to contemplate the large amounts of energy these creatures muster, how they take to the air on such tiny quantities of nutrients. Today, he may spot the little squirrel with a bent tail nudging up the lid of the feeder to get at nuts. If he's sitting here still when winter comes, after the nettles have died back, he'll have a clear view of rabbits playing.

October now, and Simon calls Jenny to say their dad's no longer able to eat. His lady friend, Beatrice, has said she'll be there with him till the end. Jenny doesn't know Beatrice well – when she and Simon visit, Beatrice tends to stay away, perhaps consciously giving them that time with their dad – but when Jenny was last visiting, Beatrice was there in the corridor, putting her key into the door of her flat, opposite. They spoke for a few minutes; Jenny became tearful, but Beatrice said, 'It will be ok, dear.' She'd already been through looking after two husbands as their lives drew to a close. Jenny sends a card, now, thanking Beatrice for everything she's doing and will do. She knows without Beatrice, her dad wouldn't be able to spend these last weeks at home.

She also sends her dad a letter. She writes that she loves him and she's been lucky to have had him as a dad. Tells him she remembers when he made her a dolls' house with working light switches, taught her algebra while waiting at the launderette, washed her feet then carried her down the stairs to tramp elderberries in a tin bath. One time, when they were gardening together, he'd buried an old hexagonal inkwell for her to find so she could dig it up like treasure. As she prepares to lose her dad, other memories and reflections come to Jenny, not all of which she puts into the letter. While growing up, her dad was off working abroad maybe half of the time. When he was home, he brought his energy, his ebullience to all sorts of projects: DIY, food-growing, beer-making. And he'd try to lead the family in discussions at the dinner table: 'So, what's your philosophy on life, Jen?' She never knew what to say. She used to hide behind a curtain of hair, and somehow feel shy to show herself even to her own family. Looking back, she'd have to say she had a lovely childhood – the apple-scrumping, the welly walks in the woods with the dog. But at the time, she couldn't wait to leave. At 19, she went off with Alex to art college. There were no mobile phones then and Jenny didn't pay much attention to her mum and dad after she left.

Jenny's work as a set builder and model maker is freelance and sporadic – when a contract comes along, she can't really afford to turn it down. When she heard her dad was no longer able to eat and was spending longer periods sleeping, she knew he didn't have much time left. He was still saying to her, 'You take the work, no need to come, I'm only lying here doing nothing.' She told him, 'Of course I'm going to come and see you,' and managed to get up there to be with him for a few days. When she arrived, to her he just looked normal, in his nice pyjamas, in his own bed and home; there was only the morphine drip in his arm to show his dying had begun. He was sitting giggling with Beatrice, and able to sip then spit out the iced water that she'd brought him. Jenny sat next to her dad, nice and close and side by side. She involuntarily began to wail – it was primordial: *this is it, I'm losing my dad.* Paul said, 'Don't cry, don't cry,' and kissed her neck, but she couldn't stop. He changed tack then and said, 'Oh, why don't you cry, Jenny? Why don't you have a cry?!' And that made her laugh. It was like *oh that's my dad, still being my dad,* because she'd always been the one stressing about something, and he'd always been the one helping her to calm down and not take everything so much to heart.

Jenny said, 'Who's the best dad?' and he answered, 'Who's the best daughter?' It still somehow felt impossible to say in person the words *I love you.* It wasn't something often said in their family. But that didn't matter now, because they both knew it already. Sun and birdsong were streaming through the window. Jenny had been worried about how to say goodbye, because she was fairly sure it really was goodbye this time. After a while though, her dad drifted off to sleep. She felt there was nothing more that needed to be said or done, so she and Alex slipped away.

Four days later, in the morning, Simon called.
      Jenny said, 'Has it happened?'
      'Dad died at 6:45 this morning.'
      They spoke for a few moments, then Jenny said, 'My throat's sort of closed up now, I can't really talk.'

In the weeks that follow, Jenny mostly feels numb, and just gets on with work. One day, though, she works herself into a sobbing state and cries out 'Sorry Dad! That I ignored you for so many years!' A friend sends her a card saying, 'You were close to him when it mattered,' and Jenny does think that is true. Another day a male blackbird comes and sits for a long time on the garden fence. Jenny notices because, with the cats that live along this road, they don't get many visits from birds. She enjoys watching this bird chatting quietly to himself; it makes her think of the painting she did of a blackbird, that her dad hung on his wall, with the painting he'd done of a cat, looking up at it. It's been nice to have a few chats on the phone with Beatrice; they are in a period of a shared state. They hardly know each other really, but they have this thing in common – Paul.

A few weeks before he died, Paul had shown Simon on a map where he wanted his ashes scattered. It was a spot on the Suffolk coast where he'd scattered his mother's ashes 20 years earlier. Jenny remembers that day – how her dad turned in a circle as he gradually let the ashes go. So, it seemed sort of poetic that they should scatter his in the same place. It hasn't turned out as simple, though, as it first seemed. That part of the coast is eroding fast, so the road Paul used to know ends far short now of where it used to go. There are 'Danger!' and 'STOP' signs warning against proceeding. Alternative approaches would require a longer walk than Alex and older relatives can manage. Jenny has wondered whether it really needs to be that exact spot; some family members have dug their heels in: 'Uncle Paul wanted to be with his mum.' They seem really to believe in some kind of hocus pocus, which to Jenny just makes everything sadder, because Paul's mum isn't there, in that field on the Suffolk coast, and he isn't going to be with her.

And now, this global pandemic has meant the pub and hotel bookings made in preparation for the day, have been cancelled. If she could call her dad now, she thinks he'd probably laugh at the absurdity of it all and say it doesn't matter about the ashes. There's a particular photograph she likes to look at. He's looking back with this wry slight smile, as if about to say something, maybe about to tell her not to worry, and just to have fun.

*

From what Paul told me of his wishes, and from what Jenny told me of his final days, I believe Paul's was a 'good' death. Death, like birth, is difficult to plan for. Yet by documenting and communicating his wishes, and with the support of loved ones and an attentive healthcare team, Paul was able to live his last chapter in the way he chose. It seems the palliative care he received kept Paul for the most part comfortable. He spent his last days peacefully, with those he loved most, and died, as he wished, in his own home.

In the UK, palliative care is often excellent. Unfortunately, a lack of funding – with only a third of hospice care in England funded by the NHS – means that high quality palliative care is not available for all. Even when available, palliative care cannot eliminate suffering at the end of life for everyone – it has its limits in the management of pain and other physical symptoms; and for many, the prospect of losing dignity and autonomy at the end of life causes psychological pain that lies beyond the reach of palliation.

We have moved forward from the paternalistic 'doctor knows best' culture of previous decades, towards a growing recognition that good healthcare should mean patient-centred care, which takes into consideration individual wishes and preferences. But one end-of-life option is becoming glaring in its absence in the UK. In a rapidly-growing number of jurisdictions – including Switzerland, the Netherlands, Belgium, Luxembourg, Germany, Canada, Italy, Colombia, Austria, Portugal, Spain, New Zealand, Australia and parts of the USA - people now have the legal option to influence the manner and timing of their own death, with medical assistance. I wanted to give voice in this book to those who are still being denied choice at the end of life - Phil Newby is among their number.

33

PHIL

speaking for those who want to live and die with dignity

It was winter, and winters are always harder. The south-facing side of the family home is a wall of glass. When you've lost the use of your legs and hands, you naturally spend more time looking out of windows than you did before. To sit here on a fine day, when you're offered up a world of light and colour, can be a lovely thing. When what you see's a winter monochrome, though – a succession of grey days – that's not great for your mood.

Last winter, Phil began to look with more intent into his options, which looked to him as bleak as bleak gets. He was on the cusp of losing the last vestiges of autonomy. To take his life at home would traumatise and could incriminate his family. He could just about still manage to get into his power wheelchair and out of the front door on his own, perhaps with pre-opened packets of pills or whatever. But he knew if he left it any longer, he wouldn't be able to do these things. The Swiss option would require him to go while still well enough to travel: well enough, then, to have living still to do. Besides, he fundamentally objects that he should have to leave his home, his country, to find compassion and dignity in dying. The third option would be to let the disease run its course.

The diagnosis came on a summer's day, an incongruity which added to the sense of the surreal. Some months prior, Phil had told his GP about a weakness in his thumb, and how the muscles in his legs would sometimes twitch all by themselves in the middle of the night. The GP ran some blood tests and said 'There's nothing wrong with you,' but Phil went back some weeks later saying 'Something's still odd.' He was the one who suggested looking into neurology and the GP said 'Why not?' Then there were months of tests for various things, and hearing they'd come back negative. Phil thought he was hearing good news; if he hadn't had his head up his backside, he might have seen what his wife Charlotte was beginning to – that with each negative test result, they were edging closer to the Bad Boys, the diagnoses no one wants to hear. It's called a 'null hypothesis' – they rule out various forms of neuropathy, different kinds of viral and bacterial infection, Lyme disease or whatever, then they rule out multiple sclerosis. At which point, if it isn't that, it only really leaves one thing.

They knew it was an important appointment. After the usual long wait, they were ushered into the consultant's room. Here's a tip: if there's a second person in the corner, with a dark beard and a polo neck, whose lanyard says something amorphous like 'hospital client services', take it as a sign this isn't going to be good news. Here is the news that summer's day, news Phil remembers almost word for word: 'We've run all the tests, there's nothing we can find to positively identify, so it's our conclusion that you have motor neurone disease syndrome.' She goes on to explain that Phil can expect to live two to three years, and outlines what's likely to happen to him, which sounds horrendous. The guy with a lanyard is a counsellor, but in Phil's memory he doesn't speak; Phil and Charlotte hardly speak. They sit in shock, then leave, drive home and sob in the car on the drive, pull themselves together enough to pick up the girls from school and go on with life.

That Sunday afternoon, Phil got a call from the consultant who was taking over, the MND specialist.

He said, 'Can you come into hospital?'

'When?'

'Well, now – as soon as possible, tonight.'

That was a shock to Phil – he was running his own business, an environmental consultancy; it's not so easy to just drop everything. But this sounded like an emergency, it sounded like 'Get here now, because you're about to die.' So he got there, and they hooked him up with two intravenous drips. The consultant came, drew round the blue curtain and re-whispered the diagnosis. Phil was lying there feeling, watching, the muscles in his shoulders, neck and torso jump and flutter.

He asked, 'What's going on?'

'Well it's amazing, it's the body trying to defeat this, but what you're seeing is the muscles dying as the nerve connections sever.'

So, Phil thought, *I'm watching myself dying from the inside.* On this six-bed neuro ward, the person next to Phil was in a coma, the person opposite had very advanced dementia. Phil was in hospital a week; he'd wake in the mornings to empty spaces. You'd ask the nurse 'What happened to that guy?' and they'd say they couldn't tell you. All this was totally bewildering for someone who a few days earlier had been trundling along with a full and busy life. As he later came to understand, this was the last bit of ruling out – a week-long intravenous treatment they were trialling. Phil came to understand, too, that he wasn't imminently dying – the sense of urgency communicated by the consultant came from wanting to grasp the rare opportunity of a vacant bed on neuro. The treatment had no impact, though; Phil's diagnosis was re-confirmed and he was sent home.

He'd say, and others he's met since would say from their own experiences, that the diagnosis could have been more sensitively handled by the medical staff. Perhaps it's how they're trained – to shoot straight between the eyes – or perhaps it's a defence they learn to protect themselves from getting swept away by other people's grief. Really, though, there's no sugar-coating MND. Phil was told to go home and sort out his affairs, get his will done, spend time with his family. He was told he could cash in his pension, because he wasn't going to reach pensionable age. He was 43, both of his parents were going strong and he still felt fairly immortal. It was hard to believe what he was being told, because basically Phil felt fine. But they said to expect a fairly rapid deterioration – MND is known as the disease of a thousand days - and that there was nothing he could do.

The news hit Phil and Charlotte with shocking force. They'd built a home together, launched a business; they were still very much in that building and growing phase of life. Their two girls were 9 and 11 – still in primary school. How do you get your head around the thought that all you've built, the life you've created with each other, is under threat of imminent destruction? That summer was a horror. Until then, like most people, Phil had assumed he and his wife would get to grow old together, that he'd one day meet his daughters' children and watch them grow, too. In those weeks after diagnosis, he'd see old couples and feel bitter envy, see grandparents with their grandkids, and be confronted with the fact that even with a very good run this was a life he could not now expect to see.

Phil is not religious. After troubled years at primary school, during which his dad left and he struggled with dyslexia, he was sent to a strongly Christian charity school, where he alternately marched and prayed for eight years. After school, he soon rejected both activities. When you're in a desperate situation and panic sets in, though, you start to grasp around for something. After the diagnosis, Phil didn't exactly pray, but there was something in him calling out for help, offering up desperate little hopes. So, when help indeed comes - from far-flung reaches of your life, even from strangers, when people offer a hand to pull you up from that dark place you've dropped down into - these people do look to you a bit like angels.

At the time of diagnosis, Phil had been gardening like a man possessed, which seemed necessary in order to keep a hold of the couple of acres of Victorian kitchen garden that is home. The fruit trees were all around 130 years old, almost at the end of life, and were beginning to collapse one after another. As his dexterity and strength began to go downhill, Phil was worrying about the garden, so it was a great relief when a chance knock on the door brought Craig into the family's life. Now he helps with the garden, and is also a wonderful companion, a friend. Another person who's been unexpectedly key for Phil he met in a gift shop in the local town. Phil had heard the Nepali owner did a bit of meditating. He popped into the shop and summoned up the courage to ask this guy, Udaya, about his hobby. He told Udaya about his problem, more than he'd meant to, in fact - it all came blurting out.

When he stopped speaking, Udaya's response was, 'Ok, well I'll come.'
'What do you mean?'
'I'll come to your house this evening and we'll begin.'

And they did. From then on, for many months, two or three evenings a week, Udaya came and taught Phil about the mind and how to calm it with yoga and meditation. That a stranger would invest so much in him was remarkable. Phil's natural reaction was to search around for ways to pay him back. But he realised that wasn't Udaya's thought process at all. Udaya had met someone who'd asked about the benefits of meditation; someone had asked for help and he could give it, and it seemed urgent, so he'd decided they'd start right away. Phil had learnt at business school the first rule of negotiation is never to give something without getting something back. When Craig and Udaya offered to help him, he started to see how transactional his life had been till then: you go out for dinner with friends and foot the bill, knowing they'll foot it next time. You lend a chainsaw to your neighbour and next week he'll let you borrow a leaf blower. But now with this disease, he's moving into a world in which there's less and less he's able to give back. Yet people still give kindness. Around the time of his diagnosis, Phil read someone saying that you don't want to be the object of other people's pity, that there's nothing more spirit-crushing. The words lodged and became a kind of internal mantra for Phil. He had to work on pushing those words out, because he came to realise he was mixing up two different things: pity and kindness. People give you kindness because they want to. Phil learnt to accept Craig's and Udaya's kindness, and he tries to accept kindness from others when it's offered, too. That there are such people willing to offer help has been a way of gaining strength.

Phil's five and a half years on from diagnosis now. Though yoga is no longer possible, he still has meditation as a part of his daily routine. He'd have to say that he's a *rubbish* meditator, one of the worst. Trying to calm that mental traffic is bloody hard and he still can't really do it. But, when you realise that most of your waking time your brain is ruminating on troubles of the past and fears of what the future holds, if you can step away from that for just a few moments, that's a good thing. He does get moments when he can glimpse a calm out there. Sometimes he can get his head into a place that's very dark – not in a bleak way, but in a way that's warm and comfortable. Around six months after the diagnosis, Phil was walking with an old friend, who suggested Phil should meditate about death. His instant reaction was *that sounds awful, that's the last thing I should do!* But Mike said, 'You should try it,' so he did. With mindfulness meditation, the idea usually is that you watch your thoughts go by without attaching to them. There's a different way of meditating though, where an idea can be like a leaf and you can let yourself go with it and drift a way down stream. Phil tried something like this; he was able to sit in quite a calm reflective state, asking himself what he thinks death is: *well, do I think I'm going to Hell? No, I don't believe in Hell. Do I believe in any kind of afterlife? Well, I'm not sure. If there is one, do I think it will be painful? No, I don't. And if there isn't any afterlife? Well, it will be nothing. Is that uncomfortable, will I be suffering? No.* To Phil's mind there are two things we really fear in life: suffering and fear itself. If you can begin to think, *well, death doesn't really involve those things,* to some degree that's comforting.

Meditation is a tool Phil uses to try to keep up mental resilience. He feels he has to be some kind of athlete every day to face this disease, to find the strength to deal with the successive losses. Nothing can take away the fact that MND is horrible. It is slowly paralysing every muscle in Phil's body. He has come to accept that MND will kill him, but some aspects of what that really *means* remain very difficult to accept. This disease takes more and more until it's taken everything: your ability to speak, to swallow, and to breathe. Phil is not afraid to admit that the thought of being stuck in his body while his wife and girls watch him starve, choke or suffocate to death does frighten him. These are things that could be involved in option three: let the disease run its course.

Last winter, the stories of Geoff Whaley and Noel Conway, two men sharing his diagnosis, hit the headlines. Geoff Whaley had totally lost the use of all four limbs and had decided he'd prefer not to experience what the last weeks or months of MND might have in store. He'd been declared of sound mind, and having passed all the checks Dignitas has in place, had been given the 'green light.' But then he and his wife received a surprise visit from two police officers, who'd got wind Ann was helping Geoff plan to end his life. (As Ann later explained to the BBC, if your husband asks you to make a phone call or make bookings on the iPad – things he can no longer do himself – you aren't going to refuse him.) After she'd been interviewed under caution by the officers, Ann found her husband – who in 52 years of marriage she'd never known to shed a tear – head in his hands, weeping with fear that he'd be stopped from accessing the compassionate and dignified end-of-life he had arranged.

That same winter, Phil was following closely, as Noel Conway fought through the courts for those who are terminally ill to have the right to a medically-assisted death. When Conway lost his Supreme Court appeal, he was told that if he wished to hasten his death, he could remove his ventilator. No one was able to tell him, though, how long it would take for him to die this way, nor whether his suffering could be fully relieved. To Phil, it seemed a brutal judgement for the UK court system to tell a man who's very ill and going to die, that he must first suffer an unknowable amount, for an unknowable duration. To say this just seemed wrong, when in other places in the world, people in a similar situation can legally choose a way to go that's quick and kind.

Before his diagnosis, if you had polled Phil in the street on the issue of assisted dying, he'd have been in favour of it being legalised; as a kneejerk, he might have supplied one of the classic lines: 'If I ever get to that stage, please take me out and shoot me,' or 'You wouldn't let a dog suffer like that.' In truth, though, he would not have given the matter much thought. But these two cases in the news, and all the discussion around them, were very real for Phil now. The thought of his wife and girls being at risk of police investigation, even criminalisation, if they in any way assisted him to die, was horrifying to Phil. Equally horrible, was the prospect of the suffering he and his family could have to endure should he see MND through to its final stages. These options were unpalatable to Phil; he was also feeling more and more strongly that the blanket ban on assisted dying in the UK is deeply cruel and wrong. The great majority of people in the UK support a change in the law on assisted dying, yet it's being blocked by a vocal minority. If, due to someone's faith they don't want the option of an assisted death themselves, that's fine by Phil, but he doesn't see why that point of view should be foisted upon all of us. When abortion and suicide were legalised in the 60s, that was a forward move, which lifted some of the strands of theocracy from our democracy. But there are still tendrils of that influence, ideas of sanctity of life, that run through our legal system - the law around assisted dying is a prime example.

It was around this time that Phil began to think, *well hang on, I could have a crack myself at changing this law.* The girls were then 14 and 16, able to understand, to *see* what life with MND meant; Phil sat them down and explained his options as he saw them, none of which looked good. He asked them, 'How would you feel if I did something to try and change this situation?' They were supportive from the word go, as was Charlotte, who was probably thinking *another of his wild goose chases.*

This wasn't the first time Phil had taken on a challenge that at first seemed to be of dubious sense. He's always liked to do what's in front of him, and when one day, 13 years back, he saw a sign saying garden for sale, it seemed a good opportunity. They were living in a small semi in town, that didn't really have a garden. They bought the land – a couple of acres that had once been a Victorian kitchen garden. When Phil launched his business and having a spare garden started looking like a luxury, Phil thought they could sell their house and build something on their land instead. He got the planner round to the garden, and the guy said, 'Ok, tell me, what have you got me here for?' When Phil said he wanted to build a house, this guy spontaneously laughed because the proposal was so ludicrous. The site, in open countryside, was subject to all kinds of special protections, for the local wildlife and the existing Victorian structures. But being told no just spurred Phil on. He reasoned if he just took the no, in the not-too-distant future, the place would be either falling down around its ears or snapped up by some rapacious developer. He just wanted to make this a place for his family to live a quiet, honest life. At this moment, Phil is sitting in his home on the spot where he stood years back with that laughing planning guy. It's a kind of cave or bunker buried in the hill. It more or less takes care of itself, storing the sun's warmth in its own thermal mass.

Phil's legal challenge asked the High Court to examine evidence from international experts, about what happens in countries where some form of assisted dying has already been legalised, and about how safeguards can operate to avoid any harm to potentially vulnerable people. Oregon was the first American state to legalise assisted dying and is somewhere the law has been safely and effectively operating for more than 20 years. In Canada, where Medical Assistance in Dying was legalised in 2016, you can see a law that's being actively policed, where any attempts to take shortcuts with the elaborate system of safeguards, are picked up.

Though Phil, like most of us, feels uncomfortable asking people for money, he saw this wasn't something he could do alone, so he set up a Crowd Justice page to fundraise for the legal costs. When there was media interest in his case he tried to get the message out clearly: it isn't that he wants to die - he's still enjoying life - but he can foresee a future point when any pleasure and value he can take in life will be eclipsed by pain and suffering. If he could be assured that he'll have the legal choice to bring his suffering to an end when that time comes, it would lift a dark cloud from the life he's living now.

With each donation, each message of support, Phil gained a stronger felt sense of the numbers of people who care about getting this cruel law changed: the hundreds upon hundreds who've seen their loved ones suffer prolonged pain and indignity at the end, or who are themselves living with the fear and pain of progressive illness. Messages said things like 'Good luck, I'm with you all the way,' 'Thank you for doing this,' and 'With love and rage.' To hear from so many hundreds of people who'd been directly affected by this law did substantiate for Phil that what he was doing was worthwhile.

He knew, though, that he was playing long odds with the case – with Noel Conway's case the judges had concluded that issues of such moral weight should be determined through parliamentary debate, and not in a court of law. Now, with Phil's own case, the judges closed ranks in reiterating this. The High Court and then the Court of Appeal refused permission for Phil's case to be heard. These were disappointing blows. Having heard from so many people 'This is what is happening to me,' or 'This is what happened to my loved one,' 'Please try to fix this,' Phil couldn't help but feel he'd let people down. At the same time though, he really meant the words of thanks he wrote to his supporters: 'You have been the tide that floated this boat.' He'd been buoyed up to have so much support from so many people he'd never even met. And he wasn't about to give up now. Many people with MND lose their voice, but Phil still has his. He remains determined to use his platform to keep people talking about the issue of assisted dying. Recently, an ITV journalist called - they were running a piece on people who'd been prosecuted after assisting a loved one to die. So Phil had a conversation with the woman who was interested in the topic, but hadn't thought about it deeply; after he'd furnished her with some of the facts, Phil thought she was more pro a change in the law than she'd been previously. Around the same time, his local MP called for a briefing on his situation so that she could speak about it in a parliamentary debate on assisted dying.

Almost without exception, the MPs who spoke that day agreed that Parliament should look properly at the case for and against the legalisation of assisted dying. Though this was a debate without a vote, and nothing was conclusively agreed, Phil felt witness to an important moment, in which he and his supporters had played a significant part. So far, he and Charlotte have chalked up nearly fifty interviews on TV, the radio and in national newspapers. These conversations feel to Phil like a useful contribution to change; if you can have these conversations as part of a normal day, that's something.

Between his first thoughts of mounting a legal case, to the case ending, a year elapsed, landing Phil back in another winter. Last year he spoke about a future point, when pain and suffering might outweigh pleasure and value. Some days, now, he feels he's reaching that tipping point. Speaking is getting harder, breathing is getting harder – these are things that up the fear quotient. Life gets ever-more exhausting – having a shower expends probably a third of Phil's energy for that day. There is the disease, and then there are all the things that happen as a result of the disease – the things that go wrong with your digestion, your joints, your bowel, your skin. Even things that Phil would never have previously put down as amongst the most awful stuff that can happen to a person – not being able to scratch an itch, say – are actually flipping horrible. Phil is grateful that interventions can be made so that his life continues to be liveable – like the wheelchair-accessible van that has arrived, and the toilet with a lifting frame built in. Without these things he wouldn't be able to get out and about, he wouldn't be able to get up off the toilet. But he has to say, gratitude is not the strongest thing he's feeling right now. He doesn't consider himself a particularly materialistic person, but he did have a nice smooth hybrid, he did have a nice bathroom; now he's got a juddering diesel van, and a bathroom that's been ripped up and left looking like a building site. Nice things they had have been replaced by things that are less nice. And there are feelings of loss and violation around that.

For a relationship, this disease is a tough road. You go from being in an equal partnership where you split the duties, to a situation where your wife has to take on nearly all the duties herself. You become an 11-and-a-quarter stone toddler for your seven-and-a-half stone wife to try and get around. You feel emasculated and pathetic, she feels worried and exhausted – the first person up at 6 in the morning, and the last to bed at 11 at night. It's hard for Phil not to resent Charlotte for having to put his socks on in the morning and it's hard for her not to resent Phil for being so bloody annoying, just always there and needing something. This is not what they signed up for, it's not the life they hoped to lead. They can both tend to catastrophise a little when new problems arise; but then they both have something in them that's positive enough, reflective enough to say 'Ok, how do we improve this? How can we make it better next time?' For the last two years they've had counselling from the local hospice, which helps. It offers a controlled and managed environment to talk things through, with a counsellor who's stuffed absolutely full of empathy.

Some days are particularly hard; he sits watching yet more rain making its way down the window, during what must surely be one of the wettest UK winters ever, and he can't get himself out of a morose state. If he were to have a long string of bad days, stretching into months, then he might begin to feel he no longer wanted to be alive. For the time being, good days - that include enough moments of pleasure and value for the day to feel worthwhile - do still come along. Sometimes there's an outing with a friend, for a coffee and a chat at the hotel up the road. Then there are his girls. They're typical teens who rarely now emerge from their rooms. If he wants to go and stand in one of their bedroom doorways to have a chat with them, he has to think now *bloody hell, that's a serious effort*. But this week he had a kind of light bulb moment with his older daughter. She's in the first year of her A levels and had been asked to write a CV as a way of starting to think about university applications. She was worrying about how best to put herself across, and Phil was able to talk things through with her, help her develop a clear framework for what she wanted to say. He's actually very interested in her studies: she taught *him* some of the finer points of the carbon cycle and RNA transcription, stuff about which he had some vague understanding, but not at the level she has. He enjoys talking to both his daughters about their studies; it's a way to keep his mind on top of things.

Though it's very hard for Phil that he can't do so much of what he used to do as a dad – he can't kayak or go running with them now – he still has a role to play for the girls emotionally and financially. He's very motivated to do what he can to put sandbags around the family's financial defences; that might not sound much fun, but it does give Phil a sense of his continuing value. After the diagnosis, Phil and Charlotte didn't rush to plan bucket list activities; what they wanted most was just to keep things as normal as possible for the girls, to keep the family's wheels on. That's still what gets Phil out of bed each day. He sees where he can still contribute, and together they get things done. The rose bushes needed pruning – Phil can no longer do that himself, but he knows how best to do it; yesterday he spent a few hours out in the garden, saying 'Please cut here, cut there,' and getting perishing cold, but at the same time getting to see red kites circling high up overhead, and gulls heading down to the edge of Rutland Water as the light faded.

An Irish friend told Phil that in the Celtic tradition, a slow death is a good one. If you're snatched away violently, suddenly, that's bad, but if you've had time to prepare and it's all gone smoothly, then the wake would be much more celebratory. Phil does feel grateful he's had time to put some things in place, to reconcile himself to what is happening. For that first period after diagnosis, he was still able to do lots of stuff, it was almost like an early retirement. When he thinks back to the prognosis he was given, of two to three years, he does feel grateful for the time he's had, the time he has still. When he was diagnosed, his girls were 9 and 11 years old; now they're 15 and 17. He's been able to be with them through those years, watch them unfurling. He's had time too, to look at what he's done in life and think, *well that was something worthwhile.* He feels as if he's living in dog years, but at least he has been able to get a few things done. Through various jobs, Phil was involved with the public, private and voluntary sectors, and he realised they all speak very different languages and have different drivers. Yet, if you want, for instance, to build a flood defence or a solar farm, you need to get all three sectors involved, and it can turn out to be an astonishingly painful and elongated process, full of distrust. The idea of Phil's business, Green Ventures, was to broker environmental initiatives: to get people together and look at all the problems, so that a way forward can be agreed by everyone. He's proud of the projects that he worked on.

Though his progressing illness meant stepping back from work, a couple of years after his diagnosis, Phil saw a chance to put his skills to use again. A friend who happens to love trees was being moved off a plot of land where he'd planted saplings and was wondering what to do with them. That was the beginning of Phil's idea to plant an area of nut trees. He had an idea for where it could happen – some spare acres in between two areas of Rutland Water's car park – and was able, still, to make the phone calls, have the site meetings, and so on, to get it done. 50 trees were planted, all different species and types. If someone doesn't come and bulldoze the whole thing, it could still be there in a couple of hundred years' time. Phil has to chuckle at himself, because he thinks of the place as Newby's Nuttery, so there's a bit of ego in there. But also, there's that sense of purpose that comes with a continuing responsibility, and there's the simple pleasure of being outside. Phil has read how seeing things grow can be helpful in coping with bereavement. The people closest to Phil are grieving because they're watching him go by degrees. Phil feels that sense of loss himself; it sits close to the surface a lot of the time, akin to having lost a dear pet or friend. The nut grove gives him the impetus to get out on his mobility scooter. All he's doing is looking at little trees, no taller now than six foot. But they're something he's helped put in place; they grow towards the future.

34

ONLY WHEN IT FEELS LIKE A GIFT

religious influence in the assisted dying debate

I first spoke to Phil Newby in January 2020, and again the following month, after he received the disappointing news that his bid for judges to look at the evidence on assisted dying had been rejected by the Court of Appeal. Phil, with remarkable resilience and generosity, has continued to campaign for a change in the law. In May of 2021, with a new assisted dying bill due its First Reading in the House of Lords, Phil spoke to Sky News. He reflected that the Covid-19 pandemic 'has brought people unexpectedly closer to death on many occasions, to their own mortality,' meaning that now is 'perhaps the ideal time for politicians to reflect on what society wants.' By that time, Phil's MND had progressed further; he needed to use a ventilator for two hours a day and feared losing the ability to talk. Phil knows that any change in the law likely won't come in time for him. But, as he told Sky, 'There will be people who go after me in this position.' He felt it was important to speak up, while he still could, in the hope that those who suffer incurably may, in the future, have the right to a compassionate and dignified death.

An overwhelming majority of people in the UK – both religious and non-religious - now support the legalisation of assisted dying. Yet a vocal minority continue to obstruct the lifting of this country's current blanket ban. Guided by their belief that God should hold the ultimate power to determine when our lives end, certain religious leaders and organisations retain undue influence in our democracy and deny us choice over the care we can receive at end-of-life.

Non-religious people don't believe our lives unfold according to any divine plan; many of us believe instead that it is our responsibility and privilege to make our lives what they are: to write our own stories. Non-religious people are particularly likely to place a high value on being able to exercise agency, and on the ability to shape the way our stories end. Though the end-of-life preferences of non-religious people is an understudied area, research carried out in Switzerland and the USA suggests being non-religious means a person is more likely to choose, or wish to have the option of, a medically-assisted death. A 2019 Populus poll found that 90% of non-religious people in the UK support a change in the law on assisted dying. It is worth noting that the same poll found 80% of religious people also support the legalisation of assisted dying. These days, in the UK, most religious people are liberal and progressive enough in their beliefs to recognise that someone who is suffering intolerably deserves compassion, and for their bodily autonomy to be respected.

Yet a key reason the voices of incurably suffering people continue to go unheeded - leaving our legislation on assisted dying out of step with the views of the British public, and with international developments - is the power that religious leaders and activists continue to hold over our increasingly-secular society. The UK Parliament automatically awards 26 seats in the House of Lords to bishops of the Church of England. These bishops can and do vote on legislation and make interventions. Humanists UK have pointed out that the 'only two sovereign states in the world to award clerics of the established religion votes in their legislatures are the UK and the Islamic Republic of Iran (a totalitarian theocracy).' When it comes to the issue of assisted dying, these influential bishops are outspoken in their views. During a House of Lords debate in 2013, the Lord Bishop of Derby asserted that life is a 'gift,' to which Baroness Flather's response was, 'life is a gift only when it feels like a gift. It stops being a gift when you are suffering and do not wish to go on.' The Archbishop of Canterbury, Justin Welby, who also holds an automatic appointment to the House of Lords, in 2014 issued a joint statement with 23 other prominent UK faith leaders, in opposition to Lord Falconer's assisted dying bill. They pronounced that 'every human life is of intrinsic value,' and that every person should be 'protected and cherished, even if, at times, they fail to cherish themselves.' Due to their personal belief in the sanctity of life, the signatories sought to deny the choice of a medically-assisted death even to individuals who are terminally ill, and who are suffering to the extent that they no longer find anything to 'cherish' in their continued existence.

Religious campaigners against assisted dying realise that a belief in the sanctity of life – that only God has the right to determine when a life should end – is held by an increasingly small minority of the British public. In order to continue to influence public opinion and decision-making on the subject of assisted dying, anti-choice activists commonly couch their objections in secular terms. Opponents to a change in the law argue that legalising assisted dying would put pressure on vulnerable people to end their lives against their wishes. Yet in the parts of the world where assisted dying is already legal in some form, these speculations have not been borne out. In 2007, a paper published in the *Journal of Medical Ethics*, analysed 20 years' worth of data from Oregon and the Netherlands, in order to address concerns within the British medical establishment that legalisation of assisted dying in the UK could lead to the abuse of people in vulnerable groups. The study looked at rates of assisted dying amongst members of potentially vulnerable groups - including the elderly, women, people with low educational status, the poor, the physically disabled or chronically ill, minors, people with psychiatric conditions including depression, and racial or ethnic minorities. Rates of assisted dying amongst members of these groups were found to be no higher than amongst the general population.

Anti-choice campaigners also contend that, if assisted dying were to become a legal option, palliative care services would worsen. However, recently-published studies carried out in Canada, Oregon and Washington found that requests to receive medical assistance in dying were not driven by a lack of access to palliative care – three quarters of patients who chose an assisted death had been receiving palliative care. Evidence suggests that, in places where assisted dying has been legalised, rather than being undermined, palliative care has actually improved. In Belgium, voluntary euthanasia (when a doctor administers life-ending drugs at a patient's request) and doctor-assisted suicide (when a doctor prescribes life-ending drugs which patients administer themselves) were both made legal in 2002. At the time, palliative care professionals there staunchly opposed the change in the law. However, in an article published in 2013, Belgian palliative care professionals acknowledged that, 'after ten years of experience,' the consequences of the introduction of euthanasia that had initially been feared 'did not materialise.' They state that 'palliative care was not harmed by the introduction of euthanasia, but on the contrary was forced to develop further. The overall feeling is that end-of-life care in general has substantially improved.' As a consequence of the change in the law, healthcare professionals and patients had become more knowledgeable about end-of-life care; more open communication about patients' options became possible; and end-of-life carers were better able to respond to patients' wishes. Similarly, Oregon Hospice Association, which initially bitterly opposed the legalisation of assisted dying, issued a statement eight years after the Death with Dignity Act was passed, in which they withdrew their opposition, acknowledging that there was 'no evidence that assisted dying undermined Oregon's end-of-life care or harmed the interests of vulnerable people.'

International experience shows how it would be possible, in the UK, for an assisted dying law to be put in place with robust safeguards which would protect vulnerable people, while also giving us all more agency to shape our final experience of life. Meanwhile, the continuing absence of such a law is exacerbating the suffering of many.

35

NATHAN AND BERNARD

a trip to Switzerland

In England, around 300 terminally ill people per year die by suicide. Because assisting suicide in any way is currently illegal, those who take their own lives often must die alone, without the knowledge or the presence of their loved ones. Attempting suicide without medical expertise leaves people at risk of facing a distressing - rather than swift and painless – end; unsuccessful attempts can leave people still alive but with their quality of life further reduced. In 2017 it was reported that every eight days on average, someone from the UK travelled to Switzerland for an assisted death at the Dignitas clinic. It is not something any of these people would feel forced to choose if assisted dying were a legal option in the UK. Accessing an assisted death abroad means expending precious time and energy overcoming logistical and bureaucratic hurdles. If loved ones help with this process, the threat of their being prosecuted for doing so adds to the anxiety and trauma of an already-difficult time. The need to be well enough to make a long journey means people may be pushed into ending their lives sooner than they would wish. The average cost of accessing an assisted death in Switzerland is £10 000, which makes it prohibitively expensive for many. The Covid-19 pandemic and associated travel restrictions have added another layer of difficulty and stress for those attempting to travel to Switzerland for an assisted death. Despite the downsides, many people who are in a financial position to do so, decide that accessing a compassionate and dignified death in Switzerland is their best available option. A few years ago, Nathan accompanied his father Bernard on this final journey.

*

Nathan was just parking up, about to meet a friend for lunch, when his dad called to say he planned to end his life in Switzerland. That was a memorable call, but, for Nathan, the news wasn't surprising. His father, Bernard, had always been a super-independent guy. He'd been something of an adventurer, travelling extensively as a political correspondent in India, Brazil, Russia and many other places. Even in retirement he was high functioning, splitting his time between London and Berlin, where he was studying philosophy at the university, and still writing books into his eighties. When Bernard was first diagnosed with prostate cancer in his late sixties, it was discovered early; he had an operation and for a long time it wasn't really an issue. Then it came back, and eventually spread everywhere. He had chemo, radiotherapy, cocktails of drugs, the destination was plain. Already, life as Bernard knew it was coming to an end. He was in pain, and the pain medication made it hard to concentrate, so there wasn't going to be another book, or any other kind of project.

Bernard and Nathan had seen how terminal cancer reaches its conclusion, with Nathan's mother, Bernard's wife. It was slow, it was relentless hours of deterioration and pain. The cancer caused huge swelling in her legs, all down her side, so that just a touch caused her to scream in pain. Bernard was quite strongly atheist – happy for others to believe what they want, but very unhappy for them to expect their beliefs to override another person's right to choose how to live and die. Bernard saw no point in going through all that slow suffering when the destination wasn't going to change.

By the time he called his son, he'd figured it out, met people, got started on the paperwork. It was a done deal. As a Swiss citizen, Bernard was able to able to access assistance to die through EXIT, a non-profit organisation based in Zurich. He didn't want Nathan implicated, but he would appreciate if his son could be there with him at the end. Nathan was supportive, but wanted to make sure his dad was sure. He'd say, 'Ok, you've got it all set up, fantastic, the option's there, you don't have to actually do it now, you can wait. As soon as you want to - three months, six months, whatever - we can go.' Bernard wasn't interested in this line of argument. He was set in his decision. Then, one of the things the Swiss clinic asked for was a letter from his doctor confirming he was terminally ill. The GP refused to write it. Bernard got panicked and upset at the thought that the plan he'd put in place could be snatched away. Nathan suggested, don't ask for any opinions, just request your medical records, they're yours. Bernard did that and the Swiss doctors were able to figure out the prognosis for themselves.

There's a process of thorough checks and balances. Someone meets with you to go through everything in detail, to confirm that you are acting with due consideration and that it is your settled wish to die. You need to have two independent doctors confirm you're terminally ill, and the final arrangements are then put in place. So, Bernard and Nathan had a few days together in a hotel room in Zurich. By that point, Bernard was hardly able to walk, and he couldn't really eat – he would just suck on wedges of orange that Nathan had cut up for him. But he could still talk. They talked about everything during those three days – growing up, travelling, maths, politics and things the two of them had done together. One of Bernard's childhood friends, Eric, was around and visited at the hotel. Mostly, though, it was father and son together in a small room and it was intense. For Nathan, it felt like a big responsibility; he wasn't sleeping well, and in the early mornings, he'd go and run around the lake a bit. Then he'd get back to his dad. Nathan was glad to be able to be there and play that role. If it had been possible to stay at home in London, though, that would have been easier, better for everyone. More family and friends would have been around, to support Bernard, and Nathan, too. Bernard was very close to Nathan's wife, Emily. It would have been nice if she could have been there at the end, but she had to stay in London with the kids.

The appointed day came. Nathan had been picturing steel and concrete, crisp white linen. Actually, the taxi took them to a little suburban house on the outskirts of the city, and in the bedroom there, the walls were orange, the duvet on the single bed was patterned, and Nathan thought *this is quite comforting, kind of like how you grew up.* Bernard seemed quite happy and engaged with the process. The attendants explained everything, got Bernard set up with a drip, and told him that whenever he was ready he could turn the tab on the stopcock to let the drug flow through.

Bernard was sitting up in bed, with Nathan and Eric there with him. The three of them chatted a bit and Nathan said, 'You don't have to do it, we could just get out of here.' His dad replied, 'No, I'm totally committed.' He turned the stopcock and he had 15, maybe 20 seconds for a few last words: he was lucky to have a great friend and a great son, he'd had a wonderful life and they shouldn't feel bad about anything, he was very satisfied. Then, it was like an off switch had been flicked. He was gone. Nathan sat with him for half an hour, but it was very obvious to him that his father wasn't in there any more.

Then they called the police, which is standard procedure for an assisted death in Switzerland. The police officer who turned up was beautiful. Eric turned to Nathan saying, 'Wow! Your dad has missed the best bit!' which, though wildly inappropriate, offered a lighter moment. The next day, there was a bit of paperwork at the town hall, a few stamps and signatures. The whole process was well-organised, efficient, and Nathan thought, *I would do this, too. Of course, it would be lovely, at 90 or so, to sit down for a nice dinner, with family, wine, laughter, then go to bed and never wake up, but that's not really one of the options on the table. For most of us, it's going to be a drawn-out decline – this cancer or that, or dementia or whatever. It's not like anyone can escape dying, but if it's possible to avoid that final time of suffering, why not?* And perhaps, when it's Nathan's time to go, by then it might also be possible to avoid the stress of travelling a long way, the stress of trying to get around the legal blocks. It might be possible to have whoever you want around you and be in your own place.

*

Until recent years, the UK medical establishment has opposed the legalisation of assisted dying here. However, in the light of mounting international evidence that assisted dying legislation can be safely enacted without causing the harm some previously feared, the views of medical professionals in the UK are evolving. In September 2021, the British Medical Association – the UK's largest medical organisation – switched from an opposed to a neutral position on the issue of assisted dying. One of the major obstacles to a change in the law here has now been removed. In other jurisdictions where the main medical body has dropped its opposition to assisted dying, a change in the law has followed soon after. At the time of writing, MPs have launched a new inquiry which will explore the arguments across the assisted dying debate, taking into account what can be learned from international experiences.

I don't know whether, in the future, I might want to choose a medically-assisted death myself. I do know I would like the option to be available to me and to everyone. In places where assisted dying is legal, for some people just knowing the option is there should they decide to take it, offers a psychologically-supportive insurance policy. Of those who discuss with a doctor their interest in the possibility of an assisted death, some will not go through with the process of obtaining a prescription for life-ending medication. Of those who have got so far as to have been given the 'green light' for a medically assisted death, a quarter do not, ultimately, use their prescription to access life-ending medication. Many people consider the possibility of an assisted death, not because they have already reached the point at which life for them is no longer worth living, but because, like Phil Newby, they fear a future when they may reach that point and yet may be forced to continue suffering against their will. Having the legal option of an assisted death could give us peace of mind, assuaging fears which would otherwise prevent us from taking any pleasure from our final experiences of life. When we know we have the agency to bring our suffering to an end should it become too much to bear, we become better able to refocus our attention on what in our lives remains pleasurable and good, better able to really *live* - rather than merely endure - life's final chapter.

36

CA125

By the middle of 2019, I was three and a half years into this project. More than sixty people had already shared with me their stories of loss and of facing their own mortality. There were still a few stories I was looking to tell which had not yet been told to me. To offer a broad and balanced range of human experience and compelled on a more personal level by the what-if scenarios that play on my mind, I wanted to include the story of a younger woman facing her own mortality. Breast cancer is a leading cause of death in women under the age of 50. I decided to reach out to women living with incurable breast cancer who may be willing to share with me their experiences and feelings. And then came the possibility that I might have cancer myself.

I had some unexplained pain and bleeding in between periods. I was sent for a scan, which was inconclusive; a second scan a month on appeared to show a lesion in my uterus – perhaps a polyp or a fibroid, I was told. Then blood tests revealed a level of CA125 above the normal range. I'd never heard of CA125 before. But I guessed the C stood for cancer. Cancer antigen 125 is a protein which can be elevated in people who have certain kinds of cancer, including cancer of the uterus lining. I was urgently referred to gynaecology and booked in for a hysteroscopy. The plan was to go in with a camera and take out anything that shouldn't be there. I accepted the reassurance there was probably nothing to worry about. I was grateful we were going to make sure.

Around this time, Michelle got in touch in response to my request to speak to younger women with breast cancer. She was about my age; like me she had young kids. She was interested in my project and wanted to make a plan to meet. I suggested some possible dates and places but then did not hear back. A few weeks later she apologised for her silence. Life had been a bit crazy. We tried again to make a plan. Then another silence.

I went to hospital for my hysteroscopy. Nervous about getting stuck in traffic, I set off early and arrived to eerily empty corridors and a waiting room of unoccupied chairs. I had the operation. They didn't find much – just an area of thickened lining. They scraped some cells and the biopsy found no evidence of any pre-cancer or cancerous changes. A second blood test showed my CA125 had dropped down to normal range. So, it seemed for me, the scare had passed.

Michelle's silence continued. I saw from her Instagram posts that her health was going downhill. And then the posts stopped too. In the end, I wasn't able to hear Michelle's story. I never had to get very far with imagining how my husband, my children would cope without me. But I think about Michelle, and about the many other younger women who have had to - are having to - face the possibility of time running out when they have so much still to do.

At the end of February 2020, Ruth contacted me offering to share her story. She'd been diagnosed with breast cancer aged 39; she was now living with a terminal diagnosis and without belief in God. We made a plan to talk at her home, about an hour's drive from mine. And then the world changed. It was scary for most people when the pandemic hit. It was particularly scary for those whose medical conditions made them extremely vulnerable to Covid. Ruth and I spoke on the phone. She told me how she was coping – how she was continuing to cope with everything life threw in her direction.

37

RUTH

choosing how to live with a killer in the room

Today is day 18. Ruth and her husband Sam were a week or so ahead of the curve in self-isolating, because Ruth's on chemotherapy. She is one of those the government meant when they said the most vulnerable shouldn't leave their homes at all for at least the next 12 weeks. Daily texts from the NHS Coronavirus service say things like 'Staying at home is the safest place for you.' In fact, that is debatable, because you have to weigh up which is likely to kill you first: the virus or the cancer.

Then there's the fact Ruth has already lost 70% of her vision as a side effect of cancer; she needs to speak to her ophthalmologist about her treatment plan. She doesn't *know* she would want to survive this crisis but be blind. For now, though, Ruth is going nowhere. Of course, this is a scary situation. Ruth is dealing with it the same way she always deals with scary stuff – by informing herself the best she can. She has several family members and friends who work in medical professions and has taken their advice. One of the challenges has been how to bring her 23-year-old daughter Hannah safely into the family home. Hannah's been at university, but everything was shutting down and everyone was going home. Hannah had been living with someone who was infected; she didn't want to put her mum at risk and said she'd spend the lockdown with her brother, Joe. But Joe's partner is an Emergency Medicine doctor, who is already dealing with her first bout of the virus and will be continually exposed. Ruth wanted

Hannah home; she had to make it clear, though, that she was taking full responsibility herself for that decision. Because if Ruth does catch this thing, Hannah needs to know it isn't her fault.

Ruth rang her medical friends, and the hospital where she's been having treatment and said, 'Ok, so how do we bring a potentially infected person safely into quarantine?' Ruth had to go to her room and stay there for four days in case Hannah should shed any virus as she moved through the house. Hannah had to change her clothes outside the house in front of the neighbours, (Ruth threatened to take photos!) come in and go directly to the shower and then her bedroom. They were warned not to let Hannah pet their two big shaggy dogs in case she transferred the virus to their coats. A couple of times, at night, Ruth's heard them padding up the stairs trying to find Hannah, and she's had to take them down again. Ruth's never been more grateful to live in a house where there's enough space to stay safely apart. Ruth's bedroom has an en-suite, and the family bathroom is at Hannah's end of the landing, so she's able to come out of her room and use that. Sam leaves her food and drink on a table outside her bedroom, then returns wearing gloves to collect the dirty dishes and take them directly to the dishwasher. There's a cricket bat across the landing to mark the point past which Hannah mustn't come. She and her mum have been able to talk at a distance. Hannah sits on the floor outside her room, and Ruth sits outside hers. Ruth can't see her daughter's face clearly, because her eyes aren't good now, but at least they can talk. Hannah's gone from the total freedom of a student house, to being shut in her childhood bedroom, with not a single whinge; she's been an absolute star. Today is Hannah's 14th day of quarantine, and no one in the house has developed any symptoms, so it looks as though they've got away with bringing her home, and tomorrow she'll be able to step across that cricket bat. Those NHS texts to the most vulnerable also tell you to 'Stay 3 steps away from others indoors,' even if those others are self-isolating with you. So, in theory, Ruth shouldn't hug her daughter once she's out of quarantine, and that's a hard ask. Ruth thinks, if Hannah has no symptoms and she's just had a shower and she's in clean clothes, it's probably ok. If Hannah goes out for a walk or somewhere though, Ruth will have to be a lot more careful when she comes back in.

If Ruth gets this thing and lands in hospital, and there are three people and one ventilator, the 61-year-old with a terminal diagnosis isn't going to win. So, when the food delivery comes this afternoon, Ruth will stay in her bedroom while Sam wipes down and puts away the perishables, and carefully gets the non-perishables to a holding zone where they'll be left untouched for three days. Ruth is supposed to stay away from the kitchen for the rest of the day, and not hug Sam, and not sleep in the same bed as him. So that's 'shielding,' and it's not an easy way to live, but they are trying to be careful, because that's all they can do. All you can ever do is that which lies in your control. If you know you're doing what you can, to some extent that's steadying.

The other term used, for what everyone is being asked to do now, is 'social distancing,' but many are pointing out that actually what is needed at a time like this is social connection and solidarity. Sam's brother Jonathan has just lost his wife; Sam feels terrible that he can't be with his brother at this time – it goes against everything. In normal circumstances, he would have been there every day, sitting Shiva – the week-long mourning period observed by close relatives in Judaism. But Jonathan has to be there all alone. They've been having Zoom Shivas. Of course, it's not the same, but it is something. Jonathan can see the faces of his four children, his grandchildren, his brother. And there has been good news too – the safe arrival of Jonathan's 5th grandchild, Ruth's great nephew. Last night around 35 family members and close friends gathered virtually for the baby blessing, and, on his 8th day of life, the little boy's name was revealed to everyone for the first time.

For Ruth, these family Zoom sessions have been additionally special because she is able to see her son. She doesn't know when they will be able to be together in person; perhaps it won't be this year. She misses him, and worries for him, because he's so exposed. Ruth is used to living with fear, less used to having to fear for those she loves. To know there's *nothing* she can do, no cunning plan, no way to take control, is difficult for Ruth. Staying regularly connected, being able to see his face, does help a little.

Lately, Ruth's phone has been ringing more than usual. She has been hearing not only from family and close friends, but also from people whom she hadn't thought of in a while, and it took her a few days to realise why. It was a little disconcerting to click that when Boris Johnson warned people they'd lose loved ones, she was the one who came to friends' minds, she was the one everyone assumed was going to die. Then again, everyone's been thinking that for years… Once Ruth got past this realisation, it has actually been nice to reconnect with people, to catch up and see how everyone is doing. Because *everybody* has a story about what's happening to them, their kids, their work – this is a new reality for everyone. At one point, Hannah asked her mum, 'Why is everybody talking about the virus *all* the time?' Ruth said, 'I think it's our way of processing, you know, most humans need to process things, and the easiest way to do that is by talking.' Ruth thinks as the weeks go by, it will become more normal, and people will need to talk about it less, because it's amazing what we can adapt to.

At the moment, there are a lot of questions – how long will this go on, how bad will things get, what will the future look like? Having to deal with that level of uncertainty, of fear, is new for a lot of people. But in some ways, this Covid-19 situation - that everyone is speaking of as unprecedented and unparalleled – isn't new to Ruth. It's not the first time she's had the rug pulled out from under her feet and had to somehow find her balance again. Like most women living with secondary breast cancer, Ruth has been looking death in the face and handling it for quite a while. She knows about living with uncertainty and about dealing with periods of isolation. It's been 16 years since a rather patronising doctor told Sam to take his wife home for a good last Christmas; 22 since her initial cancer diagnosis.

Ruth was 39 and had just stopped breastfeeding Hannah when she first noticed a slight pain in one of her breasts. She didn't take much notice, thinking it was probably a blocked milk duct. When after a while it didn't get better, she went to see her GP, who found nothing concerning - no lump, nothing unusual. After another while, with the pain getting worse not better, he referred her on. Ruth can remember sitting in the hospital waiting room, looking around at the other women, most a lot older than she was, and feeling very sad that many of them probably had breast cancer. *Aren't I lucky I've just got a blocked duct?* When her turn came to go in, Ruth didn't even have the chance to sit down before the consultant said 'Well, I'm surprised to say, it's cancer.' She didn't really hear a lot from then, because it was just like *what?!* She tuned back in at some point to hear him say her chest shape wasn't ideal for a mastectomy.

The scheduled date for the mastectomy was two weeks before the 40th birthday party Ruth had planned. In her innocence, she asked the surgeon, 'Will I be fine for that?' and he just said 'No.' So she had to ring round all her friends cancelling the party and explaining why. After that first operation, Ruth contacted her cousin in Australia – where nine of her grandfather's brothers had settled – and asked him 'How many of the family have had cancer?' It was a large number. Ruth was referred to a geneticist who suggested a second mastectomy, a hysterectomy and oophorectomy: the safest way to guard Ruth's life was to take the lot out. There were five months between the first mastectomy and that second big operation. Ruth was able to have a joint 40th and 4th birthday celebration with her son in their back garden. They were able to have a family holiday in Greece. Her favourite photo from the trip shows the kids on Sam's lap eating chocolate ice cream. When it was time to go in for her big op, she took that photo with her and displayed it on the table next to her hospital bed. Ruth has a problem with anaesthetic, so she was going to need intensive care after the operation, which wasn't available at her local hospital. The op had to be done at a hospital further from home, where no one knew her. The photo of Joe and Hannah was to tell the nurses *look, this is who I am, I have little kids, you've got to make sure I get out of here.* Ruth was damned if her kids were going to lose a parent young like she did. She still has that photo of Sam and the kids next to her bed, though they're in their 20s now, because those three have been what's kept her going through everything.

Ruth was nine when her dad died, and his death came as a total shock. It had never occurred to her to wonder why, whenever she and her sisters went out with just their dad, her mum first pinned their names and address inside their coats. His renal arteries were very narrow and one was blocked, so his blood pressure was extremely high. Surgery to attempt to fix the problem was booked in for the first week of September, to accommodate the surgeon's golfing holiday. But Ruth's dad died on the 30th of August. When he called goodbye to her as he headed out to the bridge club, she was too absorbed in The Monkees on TV to answer him. She felt very guilty about that. To this day, she likes to be sure to say goodbye to people. For a long time Ruth put a lot of angst into having not answered her dad, almost as if her saying goodbye could have made the outcome otherwise. While playing bridge, he had a brain haemorrhage, and died six hours later. He was 41.

As a young child, Ruth and her sisters were sent to Sunday School at the Reform Synagogue that her parents had joined when they married. The teachers there were stern; many of them were unsmiling Holocaust survivors. Ruth hated going and, after her father died, she just stopped. He'd been the one to whom it had been important she should go. That marked the end of her Jewish education for a while. She studied theology and ethics at A level; one of the things they looked at was the miracles described in the New Testament, and whether there could be explanations that weren't supernatural. One of the theories about the feeding of the five thousand was that there was no way people would set off on a five day trek without provisions – of course they took food with them. The miracle was getting everyone to share it round. To Ruth, that seemed logical and made much more sense. By the time she got to university, she had a solid grounding in science. She'd decided there's no superior being, things aren't ordained. People are always looking for explanations and want things to be fair, but actually things aren't; people wanting everything to be happening for a reason doesn't make it so.

As a young woman, Ruth didn't have much to do with Judaism, but her older sister was involved in the Jewish Youth Movement. Rebecca and her husband held frequent dinner parties and were always looking for a single Jewish female. Ruth found excuses to turn down most of these invitations, but about every fourth one, she'd accept. And that was how she met Sam. She never intended to marry a Jewish guy, but looking back, she's glad she did, because being part of the Jewish community has been something positive in her life. When they met, Sam was already active in the synagogue, not in a very religious way - he's a scientist and a practical man – but you can be a good Jew with no belief in God. The Rabbi used to joke that there were more people standing outside chatting during the Saturday morning service than inside praying– and that was ok. Most of the Jewish people Ruth associates with don't find God the most important part of their religion; so much of it is about community, family and supporting each other. It's good for people to belong to something; Ruth would say that's missing for a lot of people in our society, especially now that extended family tends to be geographically scattered. Sam used to be a youth leader, and he'd suggest to the teens it's actually anti-Semitism that's kept the Jews going for 5000 years, because if they hadn't had to stick together, they would probably have dispersed and integrated into whatever society they were in. Ruth thinks there's some truth in that. People find community in different ways – it doesn't have to be a religious affiliation – but there needs to be some kind of strong glue to hold a group of people together. When tough times come, belonging to a community is very reassuring; within her local Jewish community, supporting each other is just kind of a given.

Four years after the primary diagnosis, Ruth was diagnosed with secondary breast cancer. She had tumours in her spine and the doctors thought she had around six months left. Some of her friends from the local synagogue formed a group, calling themselves the JETS: Jewish Eating Talking and Supporting. These were the days before you could get anything you wanted with an online click. Each week one of the women would turn up with a home cooked meal or two, always plentiful and delicious. During one of Ruth's more intensive treatment protocols, they organised a rota for accompanying her to hospital. They've always been there when she's needed them, as she frequently has over the years.

However well supported you are, though, it's likely at some point you'll find yourself awake at 3am, alone with your fears. When Ruth learned her cancer had spread to her spine, her first instinct was to blast it with everything straight away. The metastatic team explained, 'No, we have a finite number of weapons and we need to fire them very carefully so we don't use them up too quickly.' The aim is no longer to get rid, but just to maintain. That was difficult for a while for Ruth to accept. You have to learn to live with something that is going to kill you. The question is when. Any time she's waiting for a result, of a scan, a blood test, Ruth feels that fear – what are they going to tell her? She tried to explain it to a nurse once: imagine you're sitting in the middle of a dark room, and you know somewhere in there with you, is your murderer. You don't know where they are. They might be sitting on the far side, reading a book, paying you no attention. You have no idea. When you get your result, it's like someone flicks the light on for a moment, and your murderer might be sitting with their back to you, or they might be looming right over you. That not-knowing is always a tough time. You sit with it because you have no choice. And then at some point you know more. You are told something, and sometimes it will be something you really didn't want to hear: there's been progression, the treatment isn't working. These are the jolts, the rug-pulls. Then there is not-knowing of a different kind. What's the plan? How do we move forward through this?

In *Man's Search For Meaning*, concentration camp survivor Viktor Frankl wrote that when we can't choose what happens to us, one last freedom still remains: to choose how to react, our attitude. Ruth's choice has always been to inform herself and try not to be afraid. The better informed she can get herself, the better able she is to manage her fears about a situation. Ruth has taken friends to hospital when they're having chemo, who didn't know the name of the drug they were on, let alone the dosage, and that just made no sense to Ruth. She does understand that people deal with illness differently: some would rather not know all the details, all the eventualities, they try to turn their minds to other things. For Ruth, information is empowering. Even when having information doesn't change the situation, just to understand a bit more about what's happening, and what might happen, helps Ruth feel less out of control.

To be looking back now, 16 years after being given a terminal diagnosis, gives Ruth's life a very different frame, but at the time, she accepted that she hadn't long to live. Of course, when you're told you're going to die, and you're a mum, one of the main things keeping you awake at night is how you're going to get your kids through this, how to make it so this thing that's going to take your life isn't going to mess up theirs. Joe was nine and Hannah seven at that time. Ruth didn't want her kids' memories to be of miserable Mummy, so she tried to make their days together fun. She allowed herself to stare into the abyss at 3am but not 3pm. When she was able to be more active, they'd go skating or bowling. When Ruth was less well, they'd stay at home, and play card games or Mahjong, or she'd challenge them to find an object, usually upstairs. They loved racing around, seeing who could find it first. They'd bring the object, whatever it was, perhaps a hairbrush, down to show her that they had it, then they'd have to go and put it back in its place, then come down for the name of the next thing to find. This fetch game tired the kids out, and Ruth could be with them and just sit.

Now, with a life-limiting illness herself, Ruth began to ask her mother, really for the first time, about the handling of her dad's illness and his death. Her mum said the fact that he could go at any moment was something never spoken of within the family. Ruth has come to understand that was how it was in the 1960s. Everyone said nothing and thought they were protecting each other. Ruth can't believe for a second that her father didn't know how bad things were, and she finds it very sad that he had nobody to talk with. On the day of the funeral, Ruth and her sisters weren't even told their father would be buried that day. Their aunt took them ten pin bowling. After his death, her dad was hardly mentioned. How do you process losing someone you're not allowed to speak of? Ruth pushed her feelings down for probably ten years. She's never told her mum this, but in the way she has parented, the way she's been with Sam, she has tended to do the opposite of what her mother did. There was no whispering in Ruth and Sam's home – the word cancer was spoken, the kids knew when she was having treatment, she tried to be as open as she could. She told them they could ask whatever was on their minds and she would try to answer.

Around a year after Ruth's secondary diagnosis, her mother was diagnosed with bowel cancer. It had already spread and not much could be done. Ruth learned her mother hadn't sought help until the pain got very bad; she had no doubt this was a deliberate act. At first, Ruth felt angry and let down, but she came to understand her mother's choice. Her mother had helped care for both her mother-in-law and her own mother, as each descended into the clutches of severe dementia. Her mother-in-law reverted to speaking only German and became difficult and aggressive; her own mum was unhappy in her 'hotel' and became depressed and withdrawn. Ruth's mother didn't want this ending for herself, and Ruth came to respect that.

When her mum became very ill, she moved in with Ruth. Ruth tried to arrange their chemos for the same day, so they could sit together in hospital. It was difficult to watch her mum get sicker whilst she was very sick too. It was a tough time. Ruth was watching her possible future being enacted, whilst also losing her mum. Amazing meals were still coming from the JETS; aside from that, life was quite insular. Ruth focused only on getting through the days, making her mum comfortable, and managing damage limitation for the kids. Ruth's mum was likely to die within the next few months, but Ruth did not believe that she herself would. She needed to prepare them for losing their gran, but didn't want them to think the same was going to happen to her. She explained that there is bad cancer and good cancer. Bad cancer will kill you, but good cancer won't. And here's where she had to cross her fingers – if Mummy's cancer, which was good cancer, became bad cancer, she would tell them. So, it wasn't quite the whole truth, it was the amount of truth she and Sam decided on at the time. Ruth's friend Christina also had metastatic breast cancer and did tell her kids she was going to die. Christina survived for four years. Looking at that situation, Ruth could see both sides: she could see there was value in the total honesty. Christina was there for her kids, they could talk to her about the fact she was dying. But in those four years, they were waiting for their mum to die, and they were very anxious. It's a judgement call, and everyone has to do what they think is right for their own family, their own kids. Some people would say it was wrong of Ruth and Sam not to tell their kids the whole truth; others would say they told them too much. When she looks back now, Ruth feels she handled things as best she could. If she had told them 16 years ago that she was going to die, they'd have grown up without what security they hopefully did have. As they got older, Ruth and Sam used words like secondary and metastatic; the kids began to ask more questions, and gradually gained a fuller understanding of the situation, but Ruth is glad the slight fudge got them through their junior school years.

All the while, Ruth was trying to prepare Hannah and Joe for a world without her in it. At the beginning of each term, she'd write out a chart of what they were doing each day and what they needed to take with them. She'd put it up on the kitchen wall and it would be their responsibility to check it and get their things together. Nine-year-old Joe had swimming every week. One week his best friend forgot his trunks and was made to swim in football shorts, then run around naked to dry off because he didn't have a towel. He was mortified. The next week, as they were getting in the car, Ruth saw Joe didn't have his swimming bag. She had an awful moment. She said to both kids, 'Have you checked the list, have you got everything you need?' 'Yeah yeah yeah.' Ruth dropped them off at school and spent the entire day worrying about Joe. After school each day they had a ritual: what was the best thing, what was the worst thing that happened today? Joe's worst thing was unrelated to swimming. Ruth finally asked, 'Didn't you forget your kit today?' and he said, 'Oh yeah, I had to do it in my shorts, it didn't matter.' No lesson learned there, but Ruth was relieved Joe could be so laid back. When Hannah was 11, there was a school trip for three days so the kids could get to know their new classmates. The teacher told Ruth she'd found Hannah in the dorm sorting out the other girls' duvets, because she was the only one who knew how. Ruth got them to cook a meal each once a week from when they were six or seven. Sometimes they'd moan, 'My friends don't have to do this,' but it's paid off;

as soon as Hannah's allowed out of her quarantine bedroom, she'll get onto cooking delicious dinners for her parents!

No matter how you try, you can't prepare your kids for everything. A number of times over the years things have seemed to be going along ok, then Ruth has had to be admitted to hospital as an emergency. The kids would come home from school to find she'd disappeared. They dealt with it in different ways. Hannah would always *have* to go to see her mum, even if she was only allowed in for two minutes. Joe could never face seeing his mum in hospital. Ruth would call and tell him that was fine, she understood, and 'How was your day?'

By now, these crises have happened so many times, Ruth can sort of sense people are thinking, *she'll be alright, she's always alright.* If believing this is helpful for her kids, that's fine with Ruth, but it can feel lonely sitting with the knowledge that one day she won't be alright. Ruth doesn't want to knock her friends at all – they've hung in there – but compassion fatigue is real. If one of your friends is going to die, you can go above and beyond for them for a while, but you can't do that year after year. There are ebbs and flows and planks of treatment; Ruth will be stable for a while, then there'll be progression or a setback and she can get very sick very quickly. Ruth lives at red alert pretty much all the time, but you can't expect other people to live like that, you wouldn't want them to. Sometimes, there may be a lull when Ruth feels relatively well. The alert can be downgraded to amber. But, since she knows it can never go to green, amber is almost worse, because the only place to go from there is back to red. Amber isn't a relaxing place to be for Ruth, because you're wondering, *what's going to happen next and when?* Ruth knows she can talk to Sam, she can talk to her friends, just that quite often she'll choose not to. When you've been dealing with cancer for more than 20 years, it gets a bit boring, and Ruth doesn't want to be a cancer bore.

Years ago, she was a member of a secondary breast cancer support group. It was easy to get to because it was near a station, and the facilitator was fantastic. Going to the sessions helped Ruth get used to her prognosis, and it was great to be with people who understood without her having to explain. When the facilitator retired and the group moved to a different hospital, which would have been a pain in the arse to get to, Ruth took this as her cue to stop attending. More recently she joined an online group and she was kind of lurking in the background not saying anything because she found it interesting to read what different protocols and approaches were being tried in other hospitals. Then, as she got to know people a bit from reading their posts, Ruth started answering a question here, making a suggestion there, and soon found she'd carved a role for herself as a mentor in the group. She's kind of a good luck charm when people find out she's been living with a terminal diagnosis for 16 years. Average survival at the moment for women with secondary breast cancer is something like three to five years. So, to be able to tell people she's had 16 years and she's still here, to be able to give people that hope does feel good. If a woman is about to lose her hair for the first time and is looking for advice, Ruth, who has lost her hair ten times by now, can tell her the cheapest place to get x, y, and z, or where to get the ones that last longer. If someone's fretting and Ruth can settle them by saying something that makes sense, that does feel meaningful. Ruth has always been more comfortable in the role of helper than of helpee; her field is psychology, and in her twenties and thirties she worked in mental health. When she realised she'd slipped into that mentor role in her online group she did slightly regret it, because she doesn't now feel able to ask for support herself. If she were to post something needy about her fears she thinks some people would be upset, because Ruth is meant to be the strong one.

Ruth knows she needs to see her counsellor when someone asks her how she's doing and she tells the truth – not, 'Fine, thanks,' but 'Actually…' Six years ago, Ruth began to lose her sight, as an unusual side effect of her cancer. The local blind charity sent round a mobility expert, who gave some helpful practical tips, along with a white stick. The stick had only one outing, in a busy shopping centre at Christmas time. Sam said it was hilarious, because people would see Ruth with the white stick and the crowds would just part. So they named the stick Moses, but tucked him away, never to be used again. Like the majority of people with visual impairment, Ruth wasn't totally blind; in her case, though she'd lost her peripheral vision, her central vision was fine. She found it difficult to think she could be using the stick to get across a station and into a train carriage, but then sit down and read a book. She felt she'd look a fraud. So she just coped without the stick. Because of her sight loss Ruth was offered ten counselling sessions through the NHS. She probably wouldn't have sought it out if it had not been offered; it was helpful to have someone say, 'This is a big deal.'

Ruth has continued to see her counsellor, Julie, on and off, as a paying client, and it has been good to have someone she can dump on when she needs to. One of the helpful things Julie has given her, is permission to be angry. Sam is happy Ruth has someone other than him to direct her anger at now! Once you've accepted it's ok to be angry, that your anger is justified, you can then try to come up with constructive ways to deal with it without letting it slide out in bitchy comments. When she was fitter Ruth dealt with anger physically; she'd go for a run or whack a ball at the squash court. When you're unwell and no longer physically able to burn that adrenaline off, it can be tricky. Honestly, Ruth still doesn't have the answer to that one. She doesn't write poetry, she's not good at punching a pillow, or screaming in a cupboard, because if she did she'd just be thinking *here I am screaming in a cupboard, here I am punching a pillow*...When the kids were younger she'd sometimes take them to the bottle bank and they'd smash stuff together, which was quite good and cathartic.

One of Ruth's coping strategies has always been reading. When, five years ago, she had a seizure due to a brain lesion, Ruth lost her driving licence, and there was nothing really within walking distance – at least not within the distance she was able to walk. She spent a lot of time at home alone, reading. Even now she's lost so much of her vision, she can still read on her Kindle, with the font bigger and the light brighter. These days, when she really is stuck at home, reading is her great escape. She likes to read all sorts of genres – fact, fiction and biography; she's in a local book club, and her nieces also gifted a subscription for an online book club. She gets sent a book a month and has absolutely no idea what's coming, which is great fun. You can read about all sorts of different people, living different lives. Ruth does often find herself drawn, though, to reading about people who've had difficult lives. Everyone copes in different ways with difficult stuff – Ruth doesn't think that there's a right or wrong way – you just try to find what works for you. She thinks, too, we're all evolving – what works for you this year, won't necessarily work next year, so there's always the chance that someone else can offer you a new perspective that might help you. At the moment Ruth's reading *The World I Fell Out Of*, Melanie Reid's account of breaking her neck and learning to live with being tetraplegic. Ruth has appreciated Melanie Reid's sense of the ridiculousness of life; admired her ability to adapt; and found it interesting that for Reid, work – her writing – really was her saving grace.

Before having kids, Ruth worked for Mind, in a day centre, and then trained as a bereavement counsellor. Hers was the number people would call if they wanted counselling, which became difficult once Ruth had young children. So she decided to stop work until her youngest was at school and then go back to something. By that time, though, she had cancer, and never did get back to working. As life's turned out, the kids have been Ruth's big project. They've grown up with cancer – if they'd acted out, everyone would have cut them some slack. But they're pretty grounded; they're kind and they're considerate. Ruth used to think that there were two sorts of people: there were the 'sharp shinies,' who went through life and everything washed off them and then there were the ones who'd suffered and had compassion.

Ruth's children aren't sharp shinies. They've had to go through some horrible stuff but Ruth thinks, if you asked them, they wouldn't say they've suffered too much. The kids have turned out pretty nicely, so that's something Ruth feels good about. She hasn't written anything people will read after she's gone, she hasn't created anything really, except her kids, and that's probably the only thing she's proud of: she thinks she can say she's been a good mum.

You're always too young when you lose a parent, but it would be more ok now. In Judaism, you're supposed to be buried, not cremated, and when the kids were younger, Ruth thought that would be the right thing, so the kids would have somewhere to visit her, as it were. Now that they're older, she thinks she'd rather be cremated, so they don't have to worry about tending to a grave or feel guilty that they haven't. Ruth's not ready to let go of them just yet though. A lot of her friends are becoming grandparents and she's jealous. She doesn't know if she'll get to meet her grandchildren. She didn't used to think she'd get to see her kids grow up, and she has, so it seems a little needy to then fret about not getting to see what comes next, but it would be nice to see how Joe and Hannah's stories pan out. Joe is fully launched now, financially independent, Ruth thinks he'll be fine. She worries about Hannah, about the kind of world she's graduating into. And she worries that Sam would become a hermit without her, because his social life is whatever she arranges for him. People would invite him to stuff at first; over time a lot of them would fall away. Ruth's always said to Sam, 'I'm not worried about you having an affair because I haven't arranged one for you!'

You have to laugh. You have to try to keep laughing. When she wakes in the middle of the night and can't get back to sleep, sometimes she'll put on ten minutes of Michael McIntyre on YouTube; she can rely on him to get the feel-good hormones flowing. Today is day 39, or week 6, if it no longer makes sense to count the days, now that it seems the days may stretch out longer than at first thought. When it was thought possible this Covid-19 situation could be brought under control fairly quickly, it made sense for cancer patients to consider delaying treatment for a couple of months, till it became safer to go out. As the weeks have gone on, it's become more apparent that this thing isn't going away any time soon, so it no longer makes sense to try to sit it out. Ruth's oncologist called to say her treatment should continue, which was scary at first for her to hear, but she accepted it was the right thing, and got straight onto informing herself about how best to keep safe when it was time to go to hospital. On the day, she put on two layers of clothes (so she could peel a layer off before she got back in the car to go home), gloves and two face masks. She took a photo of herself, looking a bit of a dick to be honest, and sent it round: close family only.

It's now five days since she went to hospital for chemo. Ruth has a fever and quite a lot of bone pain. It's not a great time to be experiencing flu-like symptoms, but Ruth has to remind herself this is normal for her after treatment. Today she is feeling a little better, tomorrow she expects to feel better than that. She can read. She can sit in the garden. When you're first told you're going to die, and your world shifts on its axis, the birds do suddenly sound sweeter, the flowers do look brighter. But you can't live in that heightened state for long. The tea that needs making, the laundry that needs doing, bring you back down to earth. Sometimes, though, Ruth tries to reach for that heightened sense of specialness again. Certainly, she spends more time thinking of what's good in her life, than what is not. She enjoys speaking to friends on the phone, and her book club continues to meet – virtually, for now. The JETS are still going strong, 16 years on, and have gradually morphed into a group of women who mutually support each other; they'd usually meet every month or so in someone's house, to share food and laughter. Last week, they met on Zoom, and though it was a shame about the food, there was a lot of laughter, two and a half hours flew by. The week after next, they'll do another session.

Ruth doesn't believe in heaven or reincarnation. She doesn't think homo sapiens is different from any other species in this regard. She once read a neurological explanation for why, when people are brought back from a near death experience, they often talk about the bright light and the wonderful feeling. Basically, it's the firing of neurons when you're hypoxic. When your brain is getting insufficient oxygen it'll fire off neurons and release serotonin in a desperate attempt to stimulate the body. The signals create light on your optic nerve and the serotonin makes you feel good. So your last sensations will be of a bright light and a warm fuzzy feeling. Once, a friend mentioned near death experiences and Ruth told her what she'd read. The friend was quiet for a few moments, then said 'I wish you hadn't told me that.' Ruth still feels bad about that conversation because it's not for her to take away any comfort and hope people may take from a belief there's something after. For Ruth, though, there is some comfort in the neurological explanation; it gives her cause to hope that as she dies, she will be feeling good.

Then when she's dead, she will be dead. Bits of her will carry on in her kids and be carried forward in the hearts of those who love her. She'd like to be remembered as kind; funny would be nice, too. Ruth doesn't think she's as fun as she used to be, which is a shame. It takes quite a lot of energy to be fun. But she hopes when people think of her, they'll smile, perhaps remember that, like a womble, she picked up litter everywhere she went, and tried to leave the world a little better than she found it.

38

STRANGE TIMES

on regaining balance when the earth shifts

When the pandemic hits, Ruth receives official letters and text messages telling her she needs to take the situation very seriously indeed. She's on the government's list of extremely vulnerable people. My family does not receive any letters. We're not on any lists, but I am scared.

The image of my daughter, inert on a hospital bed, oxygen prongs up her little nose, hasn't left me. In March 2020 we're nearly four years on from her hospitalisation and nothing so serious has happened since, but whenever she catches whatever cough or cold is going round school it hits her harder than it does most kids. Her temperature soars, her lips crack and bleed and she sleeps for worryingly long stretches.

And just down the road from us is my mum. For some years she's had episodes of feeling faint and dizzy, which have been getting more frequent and more serious. One morning, walking across a room, she suddenly finds herself on the floor, her neck sore, her eye socket battered. Another time, the world goes dark while she's behind the wheel and she has to hastily pull over. The cardiologist's theory is that these episodes of loss of vision and consciousness are caused by Mum's heart briefly stopping. She needs a 'reveal device,' which, inserted under the skin will record her heart's activities. As the pandemic hits, Mum's on the waiting list, the question mark about her heart unanswered.

Like Ruth, we are a week or so ahead of the curve in self-isolating. There's a confirmed case of Covid in my son's class. Though we're still being told school is the best place for our children to be, I decide otherwise. It's an unusually warm and sunny spring. The children enjoy playing together in the garden; I enjoy solo bike rides on the empty streets. Niko is pleased to get back the three hours a day he's been spending on commuting. We support Mum from a distance, making supermarket trips and calling her each day. In a way, everything is fine in our world.

I dream of being in a burning building: I manage to get the kids out, but Mum is still upstairs. I try to persuade her to jump out of the window but she won't. I dream of driving with failed brakes, of people crowded together coughing on each other, of rising floods, my daughter in the water. In waking life, I plan routes for local walks to avoid narrow paths where we might meet others coming the opposite way. I tell the kids to touch nothing – not a fence or wall or lamp post. We speak to my mum sometimes through the slats of our garden gate. I am the two metres police, shouting for everyone to 'Step back!' I don't want to kill my mum.

My conversations with Ruth are quite steadying. She is appropriately cautious but not panicking – composed enough, even at this stressful time, to generously pass her insights on. She has decades' worth of experience of getting herself through tough stuff. Even in this unexpected situation, Ruth knows she has tools she can use and the ability to pick new tools up. She arms herself with information on the virus and gets on board with Zoom. If she, living with a terminal illness can regain her balance following the rug pull of a global pandemic, I ought to be able to do the same.

I have reassuring conversations, too, with the nurse at our GP practice, who says based on my daughter's medical history, she isn't at high risk of serious illness from Covid. Our kids, in year one and reception at the time, are amongst those invited back to school from the beginning of June 2020. That feels too soon to me. But three weeks later, with case numbers falling, for the sanity of all, we send them back to school for the last few weeks of term. In late July, after school breaks up, we watch ourselves for a week for any emerging symptoms. When I'm satisfied that we're in good health we officially welcome Mum into our bubble. We hug the unhugged hugs and, as she has always done, she squeezes me half to death.

Through the first homeschool stint and the summer holidays I manage to carve a couple of hours each morning to keep moving towards the finish line with this book. But for me part of the pandemic rug-pull is the question, *do I need to tear this up and start again now that the world has changed?* So much of what people have told me about getting through the tough times of grief and illness has to do with being with other people. Going for a coffee. Going for a trip. Singing, laughing, face to face and skin to skin. But now Covid has made so much impossible for many. I want to understand a little of how inevitably tough experiences of loss and illness are being made tougher still by the need for physical distance; and how people are adapting to support each other through it all.

In the summer of 2020, I'm put in touch with Anita, who shares her experiences of working as a humanist funeral celebrant within Covid-19 restrictions. She tells me quite a lot of people are opting for direct cremation, without a ceremony. Instead, they intend to hold a memorial ceremony at a later date, when it will be possible for more of those who loved the person who has died to come together to celebrate their life. Some, though, don't want to wait to pay tribute to their loved one. In those cases, Anita works with the families to make a meaningful day, despite Covid restrictions. She would usually visit a family before the day, to sit and talk with them in their home. Holding this meeting over Zoom or on the phone instead can be tricky because you might not pick up on the nuances of communication that you would in person.

It's not *so* different though: you listen attentively and carefully build a picture up of the person who has died. For some families, it has been difficult and stressful to decide who can be invited to the cemetery or crematorium. With one of the funerals Anita led, some were so desperate to be present on the day that they said they would make the journey, just to sit in their cars in the crematorium car park and watch the webcast on their phones. It's such a human thing to want to gather round and show our support when someone is going through a big loss. To watch a ceremony on a screen is not the same, of course, but it does have some value. Anita does her best to welcome those who cannot be physically present in the room. Some have let her know afterwards that actually they felt more part of the experience than they had expected. When you cannot be in the same physical space, you can still be in the same time space, the same thought space.

The part after the ceremony is hard. People stand around a bit sort of chatting by the flowers, keeping their distance. There's that sense in the air of all the hugs you would be having now but can't. Usually, after the formal part is taken care of, people would get to relax together, raise a glass and say, 'Wasn't he a lovely guy?' But now everyone has to get in their cars and drive away and it feels all wrong, because they can't go on anywhere together afterwards.

Towards the end of 2020, I also speak again to Jane Flint. She was the first non-religious person to be employed by the NHS as a hospital chaplain, and also the first person I spoke to for this project, in late 2016. Four years on, she tells me something of what it's been like to support patients, families and staff through the pandemic, at the Leicester hospital where she works. Covid-19 has dramatically changed the way the chaplaincy team can operate. It is no longer possible simply to be a friendly face on the ward. All general ward rounds have had to cease, all regular volunteer work has stopped. As an employed member of the chaplaincy team, Jane has had training in PPE, so when a request comes in, she can get kitted out and go to see a specific patient. Her role is about being an empathetic presence. From a distance of two metres, with a mask covering your mouth, sometimes a visor too, it isn't easy. Often, she's dealing with elderly people who have some level of hearing impairment. Of course, when somebody can't hear you the natural thing to want to do is step in closer, but she can't do that. And if the person's on a bay, with just a curtain separating them from other patients, you don't want to be shouting out a private conversation to the ward. Then, of course, you don't go to sit beside the bed, there are no handshakes or gentle pats on someone's arm. You just have to try to speak slowly and clearly, and struggle through the best you can.

A big part of Jane's role during this time has been to try to ease communication between patients and their families. It is very distressing for family members to be told they can't visit a loved one who is seriously ill in hospital. With the medical staff rushed off their feet it can be difficult to get through on the ward telephone for information about what's going on. Some patients may be well enough and technologically able enough to communicate with loved ones independently. Where that hasn't been the case Jane has been able to step in to help. As a member of the chaplaincy team, Jane can't offer any kind of medical opinion. What she can offer is human interaction. Sometimes, this might mean simply standing looking through a window of a side room, then calling back to say, 'I saw your mother sleeping peacefully.' Even that minimal contact has seemed to do a lot for families, to just know that somebody outside the medical team has gone and seen their loved one there. If a patient is well enough to talk, Jane may tell him that his family love him and are thinking about him all the time, and he may ask her to send back his love to them and tell them that, although this isn't nice, of course, he's actually ok.

Jane has spent a huge amount of time this year supporting the medical staff, who have been exhausted, dealing with the trauma of having so many people dying so quickly, and also with fears for their own health and their own families. In normal circumstances, when a patient dies, the nurses would be able to spend some time with that person's partner or closest loved ones, to support them through that initial shock of grief. In this abnormal year, very often, after someone has died, the nurses have had no choice but to move straight on to the many other patients in need of urgent medical attention. Routine visits haven't been allowed during the pandemic, but when staff recognise that a patient is near the end of life they will call that person's next of kin to come and spend those last hours with their loved one. A family member who is called in to hospital as a matter of urgency may, within a few short hours, find themselves a widow, widower or orphan, and may then have to be left to deal with this alone. But if a nurse has found a moment and the presence of mind to make the phone call, Jane can come to be there with the grieving person, so that their experience can feel a little less brutal. On one occasion Jane was called to get quickly kitted out so she could go into the room where a man had just died of Covid, to be with a very upset person who had just watched her life partner die. In normal circumstances a nurse may have been able to call the woman's son, daughter, neighbour or whoever. In this case, during the first phase of the pandemic, when the tightest restrictions were in place, nobody was able to come. So Jane stayed with her, sat with this newly-widowed woman for a couple of hours until she was stable enough to get herself home. And Jane walked out to the car park - something she would never ordinarily do – to where this woman had parked a few hours earlier when her world was very different. Jane went as far as she was able to go with this woman in her grief and watched her drive away.

Another situation that sticks in Jane's mind is an elderly couple who'd been together since school, so something like 60 years or more. The man's wife had been seriously ill and was in her last hours of life. It was nothing to do with Covid – it's sometimes forgotten that people are still dying of all the things that people die of anyway. Jane was called in to be with a terribly distraught, lost person, and spent pretty much the whole day with him. She sat with him while he held his wife's hand until she died and tried to put something of him back together afterwards. You get old couples who have almost functioned as one person after so many decades together. This man was in such a state of shock he barely knew how to pick up the phone and make a call. And he felt so alone – he had no children or family round him. He did have ties to his community, but he was thinking, with Covid restrictions, that he couldn't go to anybody, couldn't be near anybody. That was terrifying for someone who had really never been alone. When you spend the day with somebody, they tell you a lot about their life, and Jane was able to remind him that he'd mentioned somebody he knew who was also on their own. She suggested the two of them could form a bubble and support each other, because that was allowed for in the rules by that point. He made the call and his friend was able to come and pick him up. So by the end of the day, Jane felt she'd helped this man to reach a calmer state, where he was able to connect with others who could continue to support him.

Jane and Anita are two amongst countless doing their best to make a very hard year a little better. Meanwhile, in October, we discover the cardiologist's hypothesis was correct. My mum's heart does sometimes stop. She needs an operation to fit a pacemaker, something that would always be a cause for nerves – added to which, the virus is still circulating, unchecked by any vaccines. Cases are creeping up now that the colder weather is driving people indoors. I take her to the hospital, and hand her over at the ward door, in exchange for a card with a number to call if I've heard nothing by a certain time. She's not allowed to have me with her. I kill time in the local town, then wait in the car as rain falls and windows steam up. In the evening I take her home, tired, battered, but this time again, ok.

39

JEFFREY

and being part of something bigger than ourselves

*'Make your interests gradually wider and more impersonal,
until bit by bit the walls of the ego recede, and your life
becomes increasingly merged in the universal life.'*

Bertrand Russell, 'How to Grow Old'

From the room where he composes, Jeffrey sees the sweep of sea cliffs laid out before him. He and his wife, Marian, had been living in Bristol when they decided to move to Lyme; part of the thinking behind the choice of this place was these cliffs. *These can be my Himalayas, my sea mountains*, Jeffrey thought. To him, climbing has always been a wondrous thing. You exert yourself physically, push yourself, and finally reach that high place where space opens out for you in its limitlessness. Some decades back, he was climbing in central Asia, and came down alone onto the Tibetan Plateau. The landscape is incredibly beautiful, but also empty. Jeffrey knew he was three or four days away from anyone or anything. He sat on a rock, and kept on sitting, and then began to feel this extraordinary sensation of dissolving into nothingness. He loved it. We are walking chemicals, and Jeffrey is fine with the thought that the constituents of which he's made will one day be released and reformed into something new.

These days Jeffrey's climbs are on a modest scale. He is eighty-five; his grandchildren insist he must live to a hundred and ten. He loves to spend time with them – it's like growing up yourself over again, you get caught up in their exuberance. But his health has not been good these last two years. Not long after having a stent put in his heart, he headed up an ascent with his son and family. They were worried and insisted that he not go on beyond a certain point. A year from then, though, they all went back to the same place and Jeffrey did make it to the summit. It almost crippled him but was immensely satisfying. Now he finds his daily sense of wonder looking out at his sea mountains, from this room where he works in his world of sound. When he gets stuck on something, he goes down, sometimes under moonlight, to the base of the cliffs and looks at the ammonite pavements beneath his feet. 199 million years ago an extinction event gathered thousands of sea creatures here and their bodies were preserved in this stratum of rock. Jeffrey contemplates these creatures' whirling forms and often, whatever was stuck in him is freed up: a solution comes to him.

He feels a kinship with his sea ancestors. Marian wants her ashes to be scattered in Suffolk, in a coastal church yard where her grandmother rests – because she was the important person of Marian's early life. Jeffrey wants half of his ashes to be with Marian's in Suffolk, but the other half to be here in Lyme with his ammonite ancestors. Like them, he's had his moment of being; an ever-extending chain of moments links them to him, in the endlessly-mutable sweep of time.

For Jeffrey it is mountains, ammonites and music that take him soaring out of himself. For someone else it may be standing before a Van Gogh sunset; or at the foot of a tree that took root around the time of the Norman conquest. We may be looking at images made on the walls of caves more than thirty thousand years ago; or up on a clear night at the great array of stars pricking the blackness. When we experience a sense of awe and wonder at something outside of ourselves, a transient sense of self-loss can occur. We feel the boundaries fall away, which in day-to-day life separate 'me' from 'not-me.' At the same time we feel an increased sense of connection to other people and our environment. During what psychologist David Yaden refers to as a self-transcendent experience (STE), we are like a falling raindrop that 'simultaneously ceases to be a single drop when it becomes part of the ocean.' A religious person may view such an intense experience of self-transcendence as a divine revelation. Yet, STEs have been recurringly reported across time periods and cultures, by those with religious beliefs and those without.

Such moments of feeling at one with The All can happen spontaneously, unbidden. However, certain practices can actively induce oceanic feelings – these practices include meditation and the ingestion of psilocybin, the psychoactive component of 'magic mushrooms.' We are only just beginning to understand what goes on in our brains when we experience feelings of self-transcendence. Yaden notes evidence from both meditation and psychedelic research that links feelings of unity to decreased activity in the parietal regions of the brain. These regions are typically associated with visualising our position in space and distinguishing between self and nonself. When our sense of being a bounded self temporarily dissolves, so too may some of our fears and anxieties. Tristan and Phil, both of whom suffer from progressive, life-shortening illnesses, have both found that meditation offers some relief from fearful rumination over what their future may bring. A New York University project, in which patients with life-threatening cancer were administered psilocybin, found that participants experienced sustained improvements in anxiety and depression, and decreased feelings of demoralisation and hopelessness. Participants' subjective experience of taking psilocybin was assessed using the Mystical Experiences Questionnaire, and it was found that those who had experienced feelings of unity and transcendence most intensely, also experienced greater alleviation of anxiety and depression. The hallucinatory effects of the drug last a matter of hours, but the comfort that comes from a sense of being connected to something bigger than ourselves can be long-lasting. Six and a half months after taking psilocybin, the majority of participants were still experiencing significantly reduced levels of depression or anxiety. Psilocybin is not yet widely available as a therapeutic treatment; despite promising results in recent studies, its status as a tightly restricted substance remains a barrier to progress with research in the area. However, a 2019 YouGov poll found that the majority of UK adults would support a change in the law to allow people with terminal illnesses to access psilocybin-assisted therapy. Psilocybin could have the potential to help alleviate end-of-life distress for many in the future; it can facilitate an experience of self-transcendence that leaves recipients more at peace with their own mortality.

Some of us may never experience intense self-transcendent moments in which we feel ourselves become unbounded and dissolve into The All. I can't say I have ever truly felt that myself. I have to tell you, when it comes to mind-altering substances, I have always been quite square. Just as I don't enjoy careening down a ski slope, I also prefer to feel in control of my brain. But reading that psilocybin can reduce death anxiety made me curious. My curiosity came up against my caution – one evening not too long ago I took 'magic' mushrooms, but a small amount. The lampshade overhead started looking extra three dimensional and drawing me up into it. I floated on the ceiling for a while. Maybe next time, I'll take more, go sailing through the stars until I come back down to earth, lastingly altered.

Psychedelic drugs aren't, of course, the only way to feel connected to something bigger than ourselves. For religious believers death may mean a leaving behind of bodies, while souls move onwards, upwards to eternity. Many non-religious people believe, instead, that death brings an end to any form of consciousness. Yet even as we near the end of life it is possible to live a story not of withdrawal and contraction but of connection and expansion. Non-religious people may not expect to experience eternity personally or consciously. Yet we can still feel a profound and enriching sense of connection to something beyond ourselves, something that will endure.

For many of us, one of the main things that helps us to come to terms with our personal mortality, is a sense of connection to younger lives that will go on beyond our own. Phil Newby and Ruth, struck by life-limiting illness at a younger age, still have children living at home in whose lives they continue to play a central role. John and Linda, whose stories we heard in earlier chapters, find a sense of value in the later chapters of their own lives through the contribution they make in the lives of grandchildren, just starting out into the wider world. I have seen my own father come to life with each grandson he's trained to roll, each granddaughter he's coaxed to take her first steps. In her memoir, *Somewhere Towards the End,* Diana Athill, who had no children and thus no grandchildren of her own, wrote that engagement with 'people who are beginning, to whom the years ahead are long and full of who knows what' can enable us to feel that 'we are not just dots at the end of thin black lines projecting into nothingness, but are parts of the broad, many-coloured river teeming with beginnings, ripenings, decayings, new beginnings.' If, as we age or become debilitated by illness, we can feel that we are still part of the great, flowing river of life, that feeling can bolster a sense of our lives as meaningful and worthwhile. Several people who spoke to me for this book told me of the pleasure they take from volunteering to help primary school children learn to read. We briefly met 82-year-old Walter back in chapter 7, when he was disappointed with a life expectancy calculator's suggestion that he should expect just four more years to live. He hopes for longer because he is still enjoying life. When he started volunteering at his local primary school, he loved walking down the corridor and hearing those high-pitched voices call out 'Hello Walter!'

When we think of loved ones who have died, we may well find it easy to name the many ways in which our lives are richer for having known that person. We take comfort from understanding they will live on in our hearts and have left their mark upon the wider world. When we face the prospect of our own mortality we may find comfort in a similar way, in the thought that there are ways in which the world will be a better place because we've been in it. In *Staring at the Sun*, existential psychiatrist Irvin Yalom wrote that, of all the ways in which he has tried to help many people to counter death anxiety and distress at the transience of life, the most powerful idea to have emerged is that of 'rippling.' When a pebble drops in a pond it sends wave-rings radiating outwards. In this way, each human life sets off 'concentric circles of influence that may affect others for years, even for generations.' When we die each of us will leave something behind of our life experience – 'some trait; some piece of wisdom, guidance, virtue, comfort that passes on to others, known or unknown.'

Many of us, when looking for where our lives have made the most profound impact, will find an answer in our closest loved ones, often in our children or our grandchildren. One woman in her eighties, when I asked whether she took comfort from the idea of living on through future generations, laughed at the suggestion - 'thank goodness my nose will continue!' But I say we can hope to pass on more than a nose! We can hope to pass on the values we hold most dear. Cancer did not allow Ruth the chance to pursue the professional career in the field of mental health that she had planned. For her, her children have been life's big project. When she sees that, though their childhood was not a smooth path, her son and daughter have grown up to be considerate and kind, Ruth is happy. For some, it is also important to leave our loved ones something tangible – a book, an ornament, a piece of furniture or jewellery that has meant something to us. Some of us may want to prepare photo albums, or write letters or cards to be read on special days that our loved ones will celebrate without us at their side. Linda told me that she has written letters in which she's tried to bundle up her life philosophy, so that her grandchildren can keep something of her. Some told me they were writing down the story of their life, or the story of their parents' lives, to pass down the generations. Some also said they planned to show their children their story as I have written it.

At the outer rings of our influence, our lives may make a difference not just to those we know and love, but also to the wider human family. Some of us may be able to look back at professional accomplishments, with the hope that our efforts and expertise in the world of work have made a positive contribution. Paul expressed the hope that some good has come out of his work as a food technologist - developing processes and packaging to reduce food spoilage. Though Phil was forced into early retirement by motor neurone disease, he is able to feel some satisfaction when he considers how, as an environmental consultant, he brought people together and helped bring worthwhile projects to fruition. Due to the risk of passing on serious infections, people with cystic fibrosis are discouraged from meeting in person, but CF sufferer Tristan reached out online to raise awareness about the condition and to offer reassurance to parents of newly-diagnosed children. It is one of the ways in which he hopes he's making a worthwhile mark upon the world.

Most non-religious people do not view illness or death as part of any plan for the greater good. But we may like the thought that some good can come from death. We may intend to leave a legacy in our will to a charitable cause. Perhaps our organs will give grateful recipients a new lease of life. Some of us choose to donate our bodies, so that the next generation of medical, dental or science students can learn from us. Some like the idea of giving our bodies back to nature, of nourishing flowers, trees and butterflies.

We mortals may find consolation in various forms of 'symbolic immortality.' Let me acknowledge now, none of us will be remembered forever. Many of us won't live to meet our great-grandchildren and they may never even know our names. The symbolic afterlife of even the very famous will last a mere blink in cosmic time. Humanist thinker Andrew Copson reflects that 'Ultimately we will come to nothing and so will everything we do and create.' Yet, he wonders whether it makes sense to 'speak of "ultimately" in the situation we find ourselves in.' Our lives are rooted in the here and now, within the networks of personal relationships that form our human communities. Unless we happen to be cosmologists or astrophysicists, we likely do not spend our days contemplating the vast – perhaps infinite – extent of the universe in time and space. Our lives happen on a more modest scale. As measured by our human scale, we can feel secure that our lives do matter.

It may seem that to raise our gaze upwards, outwards, would threaten to overwhelm us with a sense of our insignificance, and leave us shivering at the cold indifference of the universe. Each of us is just one of many billions of humans living out a handful or two of decades on this planet, which itself is a mere speck in the grand scheme. Yet, paradoxically, when faced with our smallness as measured by the universe's scale, it is possible, rather than feeling diminished, to feel, on the contrary, enlarged by a profound sense of meaning. When, for a moment, we glimpse a hint of the vastness out there, we are taken outside of our small selves, and our personal mortality may come to matter to us less. After he was diagnosed with prostate cancer, Matthew would take train trips to photograph the Southwest coast. He'd walk, and sit, alone on the cliff tops looking out upon a vast expanse of water. To feel absorbed in a sense of himself as part of the ocean, part of the sky soothed Matthew. I may not yet have been sailing in the stars, but, like Matthew and Jeffrey, I feel moved by a kind of awe and wonder when I look out across a wide vista from a high point.

In *The Power of Meaning,* Emily Esfahani Smith explores how feelings of awe and self-transcendence arouse a moral impulse: they move us to want to help and protect each other and our planet. She writes about an experiment in which staring up at two-hundred-foot-tall trees made people give their time more generously to help others. She also interviewed astronaut Jeff Ashby for her book, and recounts how, for him, the experience of viewing our planet's vulnerability in the dark expanses of space, was revelatory. National boundaries are not visible from space. Ashby realised that our lives are intertwined: what happens in any one part of our planet affects us all. In the wake of a global pandemic and the midst of a global climate emergency, it has never been more urgent that we should view our lives, our actions, as bound up with the lives of others and with the survival of life itself on this planet. We are all connected. We have a choice over what we do in the light of that understanding, and our choices matter. Being small does not mean being insignificant: our lives can and do make a contribution to the ongoing human community and to the causes we believe in.

Diana Athill wrote that 'to think our existence pointless, as atheists are supposed by some religious people to do,' would be 'absurd,' since our whole environment 'is built up of contributions' from 'the innumerable swarm of selfs preceding us, to which we ourselves are adding our grains of sand.' Non-religious people don't believe our good deeds in this life will be rewarded in another life beyond. It doesn't matter, though, because living according to that which we believe to be good is intrinsically rewarding, bringing a sense of meaning and fulfilment to our lives. And when we focus on our contribution to causes outside of ourselves, our personal mortality begins to matter less to us.

In my younger days, I would have found it troubling to view myself, as Athill suggests, as one of countless ant-like creatures moving grains of sand about. At one time, I had a notion of my words going forth and securing for me some romantic form of immortality. I suppose growing up is a process of displacing ourselves from the centre of the universe. I am 41 now, and I have moved a little further along with that process. Spending these last years speaking to people (mostly older and wiser than myself) about life, death and happiness, has helped. (If you are reading these words though, and I happen to be dead, thank you for keeping me alive in this way!) From where I am now, I can begin to understand and feel comfortable with what Athill is saying – that we are small, but we are not insignificant.

In his influential book *The Denial of Death*, Ernest Becker wrote that 'Nature has arranged it that it is impossible for man to feel "right" in any straightforward way,' because we are pulled in different directions by contradictory impulses: we are driven to stand out as individuals, but at the same time long to merge with and belong to all creation. Becker writes that religion traditionally offered some kind of solution to this dilemma, since it claims that we humans, of all life forms, are uniquely special enough to warrant personal immortality. At the same time, religion invites us to merge 'with some higher self-absorbing meaning.' Without God, Becker suggests, we modern, secular humans have 'edged ourselves into an impossible situation,' in which our inner conflict can never be resolved.

Perhaps, though, it *is* possible to hold our conflicting impulses in balance, and find our sense of 'rightness' after all? When Phil spoke to me about how he tries to cope with the fear that motor neurone disease has brought into his life, he described how meditating on the idea of his own death helped him to reach a place of calm. He described the thought of his death as like a leaf; he allowed his mind to float a little way downstream with that thought.

Let's try something like that now. You may be way ahead of me – old enough, wise enough to have talked yourself down from the insane ambitions of youth, to be untroubled by the thought of ceasing to exist. Bear with me. Go a little way with me.

We will die. People will gather to talk about us: about what we loved, what we did, and about the difference we made in their lives and in the world. We are all unique and to those whose lives we've touched, we are uniquely special. In the years that follow our death, there will be people who hold us in their hearts and speak our name aloud. There will be people who continue with projects that we began or played a part in. At some point, some decades later, the last person who knew us will die. The memory of us, the stories that made us up, will go with them. The percentage of ourselves that we may have passed on through the generations will fairly rapidly diminish – 50%, 25, 12.5, 6.25, 3.125. If we were looking down from somewhere, (though we believe we won't be) it is unlikely by this point we'd be able to distinguish the profile of our own particular nose in our descendants. We can let that be ok. We will still be in the gene pool somewhere. Some of the people that live at this point may care about some of the things we used to care about and may sometimes succeed in keeping those things going. They probably won't know about the contribution we worked hard to make during our lifetime. We can let that be ok. We don't need a bronze statue of us to stand in a public square as a mark of our accomplishments. We have lived. We will always have lived. The ring-ripples we sent out are no longer visible to the naked eye. They have smoothed back into the body of water. The organic constituents that for a cosmic moment formed us have made their way into other life forms. The world will be continuously becoming in ways we can't at this moment hope accurately to predict. Will the mysteries of human consciousness, of love, have been unravelled? Will there be an answer to the question of why there is something – all of *this* – instead of nothing? The world of the distant future will be a place we can never now imagine; but we will always have lived in, been a part of, this world. And the river flows on.

40

LAST WORDS

After the rug pull, we get up, look around at how the territory has shifted. Some whose stories you've heard earlier let me know how life looks now for them.

We left Matthew joining song with fellow cancer sufferers; having tentatively reached out to others going through something similar to him, he was feeling buoyed by a comforting sense of connection. Covid, for a time, closed his choir and his gym – his 'daily slice of heaven' – but January '21 finds Matthew being put through his paces, out in the open, by his ever-encouraging personal trainer, Max. Matthew pairs up with Carl, another of Max's clients. While Carl is training, Matthew warms up and takes Max's bike for a spin around the park, until it's his turn. They train in all weathers, and today Matthew really has to struggle with the freezing wind, but Max and Carl help spur him on, and when he's done, the three of them pick up from a nearby gelateria the most sublime coffee any of them has ever tasted.

Since we met Linda back in chapter 5, she has valued witnessing the lives of her children and grandchildren unfold over a few more years. The shock of that first lockdown hit with the letter on the mat telling her to stay indoors at all times and not let people in the house. No family visits for almost a year, and the pain of watching the plans of her seven grandchildren – in their late teens and early twenties - get blown out of the water. Gradually, everyone finds new ways of doing things. Chats on FaceTime, quizzes and celebrations via Zoom. Coming through the winter lockdown Linda and Neil create a sheltered outdoor space in their garden with patio heaters, piles of cushions and fleeces, so as to begin to welcome visitors back, because there's only so long you can go without seeing the faces of the ones you love. Still hard to say goodbye and not have a hug, though. Linda's relationships with her grandchildren have moved closer to adult to adult friendships. She is a liminal figure who can encourage and support them in their relationships with each other, before it's time for her to go. She talks with her children, Sally and Dale, about life tasks – the need to let their own children go without guilt and adjust to their new, more child-free lives. When people you love move on, amid the grief, you will discover there are things you can do which haven't been possible before. For the young ones the task is to achieve separation and independence without feeling they are responsible for their parents' wellbeing. They fan out in their own directions but still, at times, come back to the centre. There's a perfect holiday week in Southwold in the summer. Various family members, also staying nearby, gather each evening in the garden to eat together. Linda and Neil think about their lives over much shorter time frames now, holding on to each small pleasure.

We met Bob in chapter 15, on a Friday afternoon, making his usual visit to the natural burial site his wife, Vera, chose for herself. Due to the pandemic, the cemetery was closed for a long time, and Bob and his partner Lily needed to shield at home. As summer allows normal life in some ways to resume, Bob returns to the cemetery to find the wildflowers very much in evidence under Vera's beech tree. The Lady's Bedstraw and Meadow Crane's-bill are luxuriant beyond his original hopes.

Arthur and Wendy have been thankful for the motorhome they bought after their son, Ian, died. They've been getting away, safely self-contained, as often as they can. Wendy was diagnosed with breast cancer in 2018. Though she suffered with the chemo, both she and Arthur feel that all they went through with Ian eight years earlier helped them mentally to get through Wendy's illness. The treatment seems to have worked; so far Wendy seems clear and well.

We left Jenny at the point her plans for the scattering of her dad, Paul's ashes had just been undone by Covid. Finally, coming up to two years since his death, 17 members of Paul's family gather to say goodbye to him. They process across cornfields towards the sea – to that spot Paul had pointed out on the map, where he'd scattered his mother's ashes 20 years before. On the beach, they convene around a prone, bleached tree trunk, each family member resting, perching, climbing on it as Jenny gives a speech in honour of her dad. She praises the adventurous spirit and curious mind that kept him open to the world. She speaks of his kindness and positivity, repeating words he often said to her: 'Enjoy it! It's soon over!' Jenny's brother Simon scatters the ashes. There's something pleasing for Jenny in the silver of the ashes on the gold of the sand, the same fine-grained texture. There's some uncertainty over whether to cover the ashes. Someone calls out 'Don't cover them, let him fly!' which is a nice thought, but they don't fly. Dog walkers are approaching and the ashes seem to Jenny somehow vulnerable on the surface there. They reach a family decision to cover them over. Jenny's thinking *it was meant to rain today, but it hasn't*. It's a beautiful blue day. As they head back, Simon tucks a stone amongst grass in the corner of a field, so that those that know can go and find it later. On one side, he's carved his dad's initials; on the other is the name of Paul's mum - Simon and Jenny's nana. Jenny has arranged for everyone to have lunch together in a nearby farm barn. They sit to eat on hay bales and Jenny brings out the lively artworks made by her dad in later life. She has had the pleasure of these paintings but doesn't need to keep them all. She invites everyone to choose an image to remember Paul by: a pair of swans, a firework display, an autumn tree. As everyone parts ways, Jenny reflects that this has felt more meaningful than she'd expected. She has done what her dad asked of her, and given those who loved him a day to say farewell.

In the second half of 2021, Phil Newby is working on a podcast. He's calling it 'Kill Phil' - living with a life-ending illness feels like a licence to be a bit irreverent. He wants the podcast to be a serious, nuanced exploration that gives space to voices on both sides of the assisted dying debate and tries to find some common ground. He also wants to allow some space for a little light and silliness. He lets his friend and co-host know that the first present his wife Charlotte will open on Christmas morning will be a spatula – theirs is broken. He wonders why we feel the need to torture our most loved ones, but after all, if we don't stay a little bit playful, we're not being our true selves.

Lara's parents, Alison and Greg, prepare parcels for the young people who will be spending Christmas day on local mental health wards. Alison and Greg have hated Christmas without Lara, but somehow, delivering all the parcels to other young people restores (a little of) their Christmas joy. They'll definitely do it again next year and hope to extend the scheme as far as possible via friends around the UK.

Towards the end of 2021, my mother-in-law, Baba Stefka dies. She'd been living in a care home her last few years, since she'd begun to have serious falls and become confused and my father-in-law, Dyado Stoyan was no longer able to look after her. She had dementia. When the pandemic took hold in Europe, Niko and I watched on in horror as Covid ripped through Italian care homes. While we were close on hand for Mum, and my older sister was making sure Dad had everything he needed, Niko felt helpless to protect his parents from a distance of fifteen hundred miles. He had a trip booked to visit them but Bulgaria closed their borders; his flight was cancelled. Case numbers in Bulgaria were at that point low. Baba's care home acted promptly to close to visitors, which came as a relief.

As the months went on, we became less sure it was for the best for the care home doors to remain closed. Dyado was allowed to visit intermittently from October 2020. Then, in response to rising case numbers, there was another closure in early 2021. Dyado would go and hand over to a staff member at the door, fruit and other bits and pieces for Baba. When he was allowed once more to visit his wife, the change in her was shocking. She had lost a lot of weight. There were occasional sparks of engagement when she would take his hand. Mostly, she had withdrawn into silence. Niko flew out in June 2021. His mum hardly registered his presence. He tried to feed her and she would keep the mouthfuls in her mouth; she was forgetting how to chew or spit.

Many vulnerable older people have gone downhill faster than they would have done because Covid pushed them deeper into isolation. The pandemic has forced us all to think about what is most important. When should we act to safeguard life itself? And when do we say that life itself is not the thing we give the highest value? That there are things without which life no longer feels worthwhile: closeness, touch, real connection to the ones we love and to the wider world. Where do we draw the line in the sand? We each draw it differently. And when the sand shifts, we may need to draw our line in a different place.

We don't know if Baba's final landing could have been softer in other circumstances. Dementia isn't known for being kind. Pandemic restrictions and the course of the disease worked in tandem to shrink Baba into herself, away from her family and the world. When restrictions eased, Baba wasn't able to come back.

The four of us – Niko, me, the kids – fly out to Bulgaria a few days after Baba's death. We stay near Dyado's flat and Niko helps him with the paperwork of death, while I take the kids scooting around the sea park. We aren't sure where to draw our line with Dyado. He is also vulnerable, with heart problems. Though we tested negative for Covid before flying, we stick to outdoor interaction for the first few days. Then, towards the end of our trip, we visit him at home. By the time we arrive in Bulgaria, Dyado has already arranged a direct cremation. When she had been well enough to express her wishes, Baba made it clear she wanted no fuss. She never liked to be the centre of attention. The children hadn't seen their grandmother for two years. There isn't going to be a funeral, but we want them to register her death as real, to remember their bond with her was real, too. With our children, I try to speak honestly and openly about illness and death, to normalise the facts of our existence, so as to take the terror from them. We show the children the urn containing Baba's ashes.

Our six-year-old girl wants to see inside. Niko tries to take the lid off, but it appears to be somehow sealed. I conjure a mental image of Niko applying more force, the lid flying off, Baba's remains airborne across my grieving father-in-law's living room. We put the urn away and instead we show the children photos – of Baba in better days, of each of them with her. There's a picture I especially like. My daughter, aged three, is sitting with her grandmother. Baba's arm is encircling her granddaughter, offering a fork of chocolate cake. Baba's other hand hovers under my daughter's chin to catch the crumbs. But this is not a tidy business. My daughter's cheeks are smeared with chocolate. They both look very happy. After all, what is being a grandmother about, if not feeding the little ones all the chocolate cake they want?

I never knew my mother-in-law well. We didn't share enough language for deep conversation. But she gave me many things. Baba was a hoarder. She found it difficult to let go of things, but one way to let go is to give the things you have to another person. When we'd visit her during the years she was still living in her own home, she saw in me an opportunity. She gave me several gold rings with pretty stones that she no longer wore. She had stacks of material she'd bought because she liked their look or feel and would bring them out asking me to choose something I liked. She had a thick red coat made up for me which is still seeing me through winters. The last item she was keen to give me, she'd probably paid a decent sum for and proudly worn at some point. It was a fox fur, glassy eyes set in its head. She wanted to demonstrate its usefulness as a scarf by wrapping it around my neck. I shrank into the corner, raising my arms defensively above my face, exclaiming 'Ne ne ne!' So no, we didn't understand each other well, Baba and I, but she gave me many valuable things. She gave me my husband and my children.

When, aged 35, with two small babies, I began this project, I felt something of an oddity to be looking so intently at the end of life. I feel less odd now.

I am 41. More of my contemporaries are losing parents and we're seeing in the mirror that we're no longer young. It is a natural time to begin a reckoning with mortality.

Not so long ago, my dad turned 76. Upbeat over a pub lunch, he reflects that he's outlived most of his 'lifestyle peers' the ones like him who eat and drink too much and have a history of smoking. He seems more comfortable in his own skin now than he did when we were both younger. He tells me his life insurers have let him know that at the point he reaches 82, he'll have paid more money into the policy than will be paid out. He's taken it as a kind of compliment: if they're betting on him reaching 82, he jolly well intends to do so. Not so long ago, my Mum caught Covid. This was what we'd spent two years fearing. But she's triple vaxxed and she got through it. A week after Mum, Dyado fifteen hundred miles away, got Covid, too. He also came through it ok. I am thankful for the human ingenuity that has protected them and so many others.

Soon after Baba's death, after we had come back home, Niko and I were lying together in the dark and he asked me about what my parents want. My dad, like Baba, wants a direct cremation – no service – but he wants a family knees up afterwards. My mum wants to be buried and for a tree to be planted in her memory – maybe a copper beech or silver birch.

'Do you know what I want?' I ask.
'Not to die!' My husband knows me well.

When I set out to find people who have been through, and are going through, very tough times, somewhere inside me was a child wanting to be told that somehow everything is really ok, and will always be ok. But there is a certain brutality to a non-religious worldview. Seeing the world without the lens of faith, we recognise there can be no easy answers. Sometimes it's nice to curl up with the kids and watch a film. If they get scared, I can reassure them children's films always have a happy ending. We – you and I – aren't children. We can't believe in happy endings in any straightforward, simple way.

Not everything is ok. Some things, sometimes, can be made more so. When we look up and see a rainbow, a robin or an ancient tree. When we look back at all the good times, and at all that's still good in our lives right now. When we look around us and see people that we love. When we feel the warmth of sunshine or a hug. I am so grateful to have met the people that I met, and to have had the conversations I have had, during the course of working on this book. The whole experience has helped me feel a deep sense of being part of our human family. Even when there are no easy answers, it helps to know we're grappling with the questions together. I have always found reading a book to be a good way of feeling close to others. Writing this book, I have felt that warmth of closeness, too. Above all, *we* are what make each other's lives – from the beginning of the story to its end – as happy as can be.

If you liked this book I would really appreciate a short review. Reviews make a great difference in helping readers find books. Many thanks for your help in spreading the word!

ABOUT THE AUTHOR

Valerie Jack is a writer and former teacher. Following developmental work with the National Theatre Studio and Hampstead Theatre, her play, *Fireworks* was staged in London twice. Her poetry has been widely published, including in the *Times Literary Supplement* and *The Spectator*. Her first poetry collection, *Educational*, was published by tall-lighthouse in 2009. More recent poems, begun while she was living aboard a narrowboat, explore lives lived on, next to and under water. These days, she lives on dry land in Buckinghamshire, England, with her husband and children, and is working on her first novel.

ACKNOWLEDGEMENTS

Thank you

to my sisters and parents who have been my most consistent cheerleaders over the years. Thank you for reading, commenting, believing.

to my brother-in-law Chris, whose insights pointed me in the right direction.

to my friends who've read parts or versions of this book at various stages and whose thoughts and encouragement lifted me forward. Thank you to Anthony, Kirsty, Anna, Jessie, Kiran, Martyn, Emily, Gabriel, Siobhan and Christopher.

to Humanists UK, the Association of Black Humanists, MET UP UK, the Younger Breast Cancer Network UK, the Council of Ex-Muslims of Britain and Child Bereavement UK, who helped me spread the word in my search for participants.

to Trevor Moore of My Death, My Decision, who championed this project from its early stages and throughout.

to my agent Tom Drake-Lee whose investment of time and energy made this a better book.

to my editor Liz Houghton for her astute notes.

to my husband whose unwavering support in every way made this book possible and to my children who are my hope, my joy, my meaning.

to all who so generously entrusted me with your stories. Meeting you and hearing what you had to say has made my life immeasurably richer. Thank you so much.

NOTES

1 Beginning at the End

2021 British Social Attitudes survey: information retrieved from
https://bsa.natcen.ac.uk/media/39293/1_bsa36_religion.pdf on 2 July
2020 and https://humanism.org.uk/2021/04/01/latest-british-social-
attitudes-survey-shows-huge-generational-surge-in-the-non-religious/ on 16
July 2021.
a humanist is someone who: retrieved from
https://humanists.uk/humanism/ on 28 September 2021.
According to research published by Co-op Funeralcare: information
retrieved from https://www.co-operative.coop/media/news-
releases/coronavirus-pandemic-helps-twenty-four-million-adults-become-
more-compassionate on 29 September 2021.

3 Jane *and non-religious pastoral support, i*

nearly half of us in the UK die in hospital: Public Health England
figures retrieved from https://fingertips.phe.org.uk/profile/end-of-
life/data#page/0 on 15 February 2019.
When the NHS was established in 1948: Information on the history of
chaplaincy in the NHS retrieved from
https://www.cuh.nhs.uk/chaplaincy/history-chaplaincy on 15 February
2019.
In 2015, NHS England released guidelines: retrieved from nhs-
chaplaincy-guidelines-2015.pdf (england.nhs.uk) on 1 January 2021.

A 2017 poll found: retrieved from https://humanism.org.uk/wp-content/uploads/Humanists-UK-polling-on-pastoral-care-in-the-UK.pdf on 15 September 2020.

4 John: *here and now, reality is sufficient*

Thomas Hardy wrote about the 'family face,': in his poem 'Heredity.'

7 A Fear Brewed in The Guts *and how secular philosophy may or may not help*

The relationship between religiosity and death anxiety: Jonathan Jong, Robert Ross, Tristan Philip, Si-Hua Chang, Naomi Simons &Jamin Halberstadt, 'The religious correlates of death anxiety: a systematic review and meta-analysis,' *Religion, Brain & Behavior*, 2017.
Richard Dawkins, on his scale of belief and unbelief: Richard Dawkins, *The God Delusion,* (Black Swan, 2007) p73.
Dale McGowan, writer and speaker on non-religious parenting: Dale McGowan, Molleen Matsumura, Amanda Metskas and Jan Devor, *Raising Freethinkers,* (AMACOM books, 2009); Chapter Seven, Dale McGowan 'Death and Life,' pp 175-177.
As humanist philosopher Peter Cave observes: Andrew Copson and A.C. Grayling ed., *The Wiley Blackwell Handbook of Humanism,* (Wiley Blackwell, 2015); Peter Cave essay, 'Death as Annihilation,' p76.
'symmetry argument,': Lucretius, *De Rerum Natura*, available in many translations.
I had been dead for billions and billions of years: Mark Twain quotation retrieved from https://www.goodreads.com/quotes/25647-i-do-not-fear-death-i-had-been-dead-for on 28 December 2020.
each of us experiences only life: A.C. Grayling, *The Meaning of Things* (Phoenix, 2002), p30.
The Ancient Greek philosopher Epicurus: Epicurus, 'Letter to Menoeceus', available in many translations.
non-religious memoirist Diana Athill: Diana Athill, *Alive, Alive, Oh!* (Granta, 2015), p156 and p161.
In conversation with Robert McCrum: Robert McCrum, *Every Third Thought,* (Picador, 2017), p150.

10 On Joining Song: *secular community and connection*

no significant correlation between religiosity and happiness: Liesbeth

Snoop, 'Religiousness and happiness in three nations: a research note,' *Journal of Happiness Studies,* 9, pp. 207–211 (2008).

Roy Speckhardt, executive director of the American Humanist Association: retrieved from https://thehumanist.com/news/religion/ignorance-bliss-religious-people-seem-happier-nones on 1 January 2021.

a subsequent study involving 26 countries: retrieved from https://www.pewforum.org/2019/01/31/religions-relationship-to-happiness-civic-engagement-and-health-around-the-world/ on 1 January 2021.

today, only 18% of people: information retrieved from https://www.bsa.natcen.ac.uk/media/39293/1_bsa36_religion.pdf on 4 September 2020.

chronic illnesses, such as cancer: Helgeson VS, Cohen S. Social support and adjustment to cancer: Reconciling descriptive, correlational, and intervention research. Health Psychology. 1996;15:135–148.

coronary heart disease: Uchino BN, Cacioppo JT, Kiecolt Glaser KG. The relationships between social support and physiological processes: A review with emphasis on underlying mechanisms and implications for health. Psychological Bulletin. 1996;119:488–531.

and diabetes: Cheng TYL, Boey KW. Coping, social support, and depressive symptoms of older adults with type II Diabetes Mellitus. Clinical Gerontologist. 2000;22:15–30.

loneliness is associated with: Holt-Lunstad, J., Smith, T. B., Baker, M., Harris, T., & Stephenson, D. (2015). Loneliness and social isolation as risk factors for mortality: A meta-analytic review. Perspectives on Psychological Science, 10, 227-237.

inspired him to bring people together to celebrate life: Comments made during Sunday Assembly: Grief, 20th May 2018, at Conway Hall, London.

Sunday Assembly should be a place of compassion: Information retrieved from https://sundayassembly.online/about-sunday-assembly/ on 15 September 2020.

Singing together can forge rapid bonds: Eiluned Pearce, Jacques Launay and Robin I. M. Dunbar, 'The ice-breaker effect: singing mediates fast social bonding,' *Royal Society Open Science,* October 2015, volume 2, issue 10.

can help alleviate anxiety and depression: Daisy Fancourt, Aaron Williamon, Livia A Carvalho, Andrew Steptoe, Rosie Dow and Ian Lewis, 'Singing modulates mood, stress, cortisol, cytokine and neuropeptide activity in cancer patients and carers,' ecancer 10 631 (2016).

how comforting it is to see all those other lights: Irvin Yalom, *Staring at the Sun,* (Piatkus, 2011), p180.

11 Someone at Your Bedside *and non-religious pastoral support, ii*

Lindsay van Dijk became the first humanist: retrieved from
https://humanism.org.uk/2019/03/19/the-art-of-listening-an-interview-
with-humanist-pastoral-carer-lindsay-van-dijk/ on 15 September 2020.

12 Margaret *and non-religious funerals*

a report published by Co-operative Funeralcare: 'Burying Traditions:
The Changing Face of UK Funerals,' p2,3,18, retrieved from
https://assets.ctfassets.net/iqbixcpmwym2/5v6n2gA1yGR5BCDRJ4kNKu
/93696c8e8e2f9e260795c941fa96c6c9/3876_1_Funeralcare_Media_pack_a
rtwork_SML_v4.pdf on 31 January 2020.
Words such as: quotations from 'Afterglow' by Helen Lowrie Marshall;
'Farewell my Friends' by Rabindranath Tagore; and 'He is Gone' by David
Harkins.

15 Bob *and his search for meaning in a living place*

Hobgoblin, nor foul fiend: Christopher Reid, *A Scattering,* (Areté Books,
2009), 'The Unfinished', 5, p27.
Since the first woodland burial ground in the UK: Information
retrieved from http://www.naturaldeath.org.uk/index.php?page=the-anbg
on 22 May 2020.
Though a definition for natural burial: information retrieved from
Andrew Copson and A.C. Grayling ed., *The Wiley Blackwell Handbook of
Humanism,* Ken Warpole 'Making a Home in this World: Humanism and
Architecture' p206 (Wiley Blackwell, London, 2015).

16 An Ongoing Search for Meaning

**compared outcomes amongst bereaved religious believers and
atheists:** Jacob S. Sawyer and Melanie E. Brewster, 'Assessing
posttraumatic growth, complicated grief, and psychological distress in
bereaved atheists and believers,' *Death Studies*, 2018, p8, retrieved from
DOI: 10.1080/07481187.2018.1446061 on 15 February 2019.
However, research shows that non-religious people: David Speed,
Thomas J. Coleman III, and Joseph Langston, 'What do you mean,"What
does it all mean?" Atheism, nonreligion, and life meaning.' *Sage Open* 8, no.
1 (2018): 2158244017754238.

17 Roger *and the treasure chest of memories*

'symbolic immortality': A term first coined by psychiatrist Robert J. Lifton in Living and Dying (Praeger, New York, 1974).
Humanist author Arthur Dobrin: Retrieved from https://arthurdobrin.files.wordpress.com/2010/09/love_stronger_than_de ath.pdf on 22 May 2020.
Ann Druyan expressed a similar sentiment: Ann Druyan, 'Ann Druyan Talks About Science, Religion, Wonder, Awe...And Carl Sagan', Skeptical Inquirer, Volume 27.6, November/December 2003, retrieved from https://www.csicop.org/si/show/ann_druyan_talks_about_science_religio n on 13 February 2019.

19 Claire *and secular support when a baby dies*

In the UK, around 15 babies die: information retrieved from https://www.sands.org.uk/our-work/baby-death-current-picture/how-many-babies-die on 15 February 2019.
non-religious baby funerals: David Savage, *Non-Religious Pastoral Care: A Practical Guide*, (Routledge, 2019), p95; Savage references the British Social Attitudes survey of 2017, which found that 61% of people aged 25-34, and 56% of people aged 34-44 are non-religious.
Since the latest information shows: information retrieved from https://humanists.uk/2021/04/01/latest-british-social-attitudes-survey-shows-huge-generational-surge-in-the-non-religious/ on 1 October 2021.
However, worryingly, in only 14% of cases: 'Audit of Bereavement Care Provision in UK Neonatal Units 2018,' p3, retrieved from https://www.sands.org.uk/audit-bereavement-care-provision-uk-neonatal-units-2018 on 3 February 2020.

21 11:11 and Other Moments in Time

a Jon Ronson podcast episode: 'Jon Ronson On,' Series 7, episode 1, '11:11,' retrieved from https://www.bbc.co.uk/programmes/b01rlrjz on 30 March 2022.

22 Alison: *just because you haven't seen a unicorn...*

For Greg, it helped to remember that Lara's energy hasn't died: The words of National Public Radio commentator Aaron Freeman, sometimes referred to as 'Why You Want a Physicist to Speak at Your Funeral' were originally broadcast as part of the NPR news programme All Things

Considered, as the segment 'Planning Ahead Can Make a Difference in the End,' recording and transcript retrieved from https://www.npr.org/templates/story/story.php?storyId=4675953?storyId=4675953&t=1550059790374 on 13 February 2019.

Reading about bereavement: Brook Noel and Pamela D. Blair, *I Wasn't Ready to Say Goodbye* (Sourcebooks, Inc., 2008); Sara Ryan, *Justice for Laughing Boy: Connor Sparrowhawk - a Death by Indifference,* (Jessica Kingsley Publishers, 2017.)

23 In Our Hearts and in The World

most rituals were a unique reflection: Michael Norton and Francesca Gino, 'Rituals Alleviate Grieving for Loved Ones, Lovers, and Lotteries.' *Journal of Experimental Psychology: General,* 143, 266-272. (2014)

24 Sophie: *going through the big stuff young*

Motherless Daughters: Hope Edelman, *Motherless Daughters,* (Addison-Wesley, 1994.)

26 The Nature Prescription

Walking in a forest: Juyoung Lee, Yuko Tsunetsugu, Norimasa Takayama, et al., "Influence of Forest Therapy on Cardiovascular Relaxation in Young Adults," Evidence-Based Complementary and Alternative Medicine, vol. 2014, Article ID 834360, 7 pages, 2014. https://doi.org/10.1155/2014/834360. Retrieved on 13 February 2019.

When we walk in nature: Gregory N. Bratman, J. Paul Hamilton, Kevin S. Hahn, Gretchen C. Daily, and James J. Gross, 'Nature experience reduces rumination and subgenual prefrontal cortex activation', PNAS July 14, 2015 112 (28) 8567-8572; published ahead of print June 29, 2015 https://doi.org/10.1073/pnas.1510459112, retrieved on 13 February 2019.

Studies show that people find blue spaces: Mathew White, Amanda Smith, Kelly Humphryes, Sabine Pahl, Deborah Snelling, Michael Depledge, 'Blue space: The importance of water for preference, affect, and restorativeness ratings of natural and built scenes,' *Journal of Environmental Psychology*, Volume 30, Issue 4, December 2010, pp. 482-493.

27 Diana and Bridget *and good that comes from loss*

the term posttraumatic growth: Information retrieved from https://ptgi.uncc.edu/what-is-ptg/ on 30 June 2020.

Posttraumatic Growth Inventory: Retrieved from
https://results.wa.gov/sites/default/files/WendyFraser_Oct28_HANDO
UT.pdf on 30 March 2022.
those who have experienced severe adversity: Daniel Lim and David
DeSteno, 'Suffering and compassion: the links among adverse life
experiences, empathy, compassion, and pro-social behaviour' *Emotion*, 16
(2016) pp175-72.
'a bit like turning shit into fertiliser.': Mark Longley's podcast 'Death: A
Podcast about love, grief & hope,' retrieved from
https://podcasts.apple.com/nz/podcast/death-love-grief-and-
hope/id1466192622 on 1 June 2020.

29 Tristan

Studies have shown that people with CF: Alexandra L Quittner, Lutz
Goldbeck, Janice Abbott, Alistair Duff, Patrick Lambrecht, Amparo Solé,
Marijke M Tibosch, Agneta Bergsten Brucefors, Hasan Yüksel, Paola
Catastini, Laura Blackwell, Dave Barker, 'Prevalence of depression and
anxiety in patients with cystic fibrosis and parent caregivers: results of The
International Depression Epidemiological Study across nine countries,'
Thorax, 2014;69:1090-1097. doi:10.1136/thoraxjnl-2014-205983.

30 Before I Die…*and the death awareness movement*

the average baby boy was not expected to reach his 41st Retrieved from
https://www.ons.gov.uk/peoplepopulationandcommunity/birthsdeathsand
marriages/lifeexpectancies/articles/howhaslifeexpectancychangedovertime
/2015-09-09 on 10 August 2020.
dramatic increases in life expectancy: Retrieved from
https://www.ons.gov.uk/peoplepopulationandcommunity/birthsdeathsand
marriages/lifeexpectancies/bulletins/nationallifetablesunitedkingdom/latest
on 10 August 2020.
Death Café: retrieved from https://deathcafe.com/what/ on 11 August
2020.
Candy Chang's 'Before I Die' project: retrieved from
https://beforeidieproject.com/story on 11 August 2020.

31 Flipping the Story: *the days on which we live*

Our brains have a negativity bias: Miriam Akhtar, *What is Post-Traumatic
Growth?* (Watkins, 2017) p109.
life **as the giddy exception:** McGowan, p192-193.
lower levels of death anxiety amongst older adults: Rosanna W.L. Lau

and Sheung-Tak Cheng, 'Gratitude Lessens Death Anxiety,' *European Journal of Ageing* volume 8, Article number: 169 (2011).

higher levels of subjective well-being: Shane J. Sacco, Crystal L. Park, D.P. Suresh, and Deborah Bliss, 'Living with heart failure: Psychosocial resources, meaning, gratitude and well-being,' *Heart & Lung*, Volume 43, Issue 3, May–June 2014, Pages 213-218.

effective ways to boost well-being: Alex M. Wood, Jeffrey J. Froh, Adam W. A. Geraghty, 'Gratitude and well-being: A review and theoretical integration,' *Clinical Psychology Review*, Volume 30, Issue 7, November 2010, pp. 890-905.

33 Phil: *speaking for those who want to live and die with dignity*

As Ann later explained to the BBC:
https://www.bbc.co.uk/news/av/uk-47152752/assisted-dying-i-just-wish-the-law-would-allow-me-to-have-him-for-a-little-longer accessed on 4 March 2020.

34 Only When it Feels Like a Gift: *religious influence in the assisted dying debate*

Phil spoke to Sky News: Retrieved from
https://news.sky.com/story/assisted-dying-it-might-be-too-late-for-me-but-i-want-it-for-those-who-come-after-me-12317078 on 23 September 2021.

A 2019 Populus poll: Retrieved from
https://yonderconsulting.com/poll/dignity-in-dying/ on 23 September 2021.

Humanists UK have pointed out that: Retrieved from
https://humanism.org.uk/campaigns/secularism/constitutional-reform/bishops-in-the-lords/ on 19 October 2020.

life is a gift only when it feels like a gift: Retrieved from
https://www.dignityindying.org.uk/blog-post/members-house-lords-debate-assisted-dying/ on 19 October 2020.

they fail to cherish themselves: Retrieved from
https://www.cbcew.org.uk/assisted-dying-bill-faith-leaders-statement/ on 19 October 2020.

no higher than amongst the general population: Margaret P Battin, Agnes van der Heide, Linda Ganzini, Gerrit van der Wal, Bregje D Onwuteaka-Philipsen, 'Legal physician-assisted dying in Oregon and the Netherlands: evidence concerning the impact on patients in "vulnerable" groups,' *Journal of Medical Ethics* 2007;33:591-597.

three quarters of patients who chose an assisted death had been receiving palliative care: James Downar, Robert A. Fowler, Roxanne

Halko, Larkin Davenport Huyer, Andrea D. Hill and Jennifer L. Gibson, 'Early experience with medical assistance in dying in Ontario, Canada: a cohort study,' *Canadian Medical Association Journal,* February 24, 2020 192 (8) E173-E181; Luai Al Rabadi, Michael LeBlanc, Taylor Bucy, Lee M. Ellis, Dawn L. Hershman, Frank L. Meyskens Jr, Lynne Taylor, Charles D. Blanke, 'Trends in Medical Aid in Dying in Oregon and Washington,' August 9, 2019. doi:10.1001/jamanetworkopen.2019.8648.

end-of-life care in general has substantially improved: Paul Vanden Berghe, Arsène Mullíe, Marc Desmet and Gert Huysman, 'Assisted dying - the current
situation in Flanders: euthanasia embedded in palliative care,' *European Journal of Palliative Care,* 20(6):266-272.

no evidence that assisted dying undermined Oregon's end-of-life care: retrieved from
https://www.theguardian.com/commentisfree/2014/jul/02/legalise-assisted-dying-professor-john-ashton-bill on 22 October 2010.

35 Nathan and Bernard: *a trip to Switzerland*

around 300 terminally ill people per year die by suicide: Information retrieved from https://cdn.dignityindying.org.uk/wp-content/uploads/Research_FOI_Suicides.pdf on 23 October 2020.
In 2017 it was reported that every eight days on average: Information retrieved from https://features.dignityindying.org.uk/true-cost-dignitas/ on 24 October 2020.

37 Ruth: *choosing how to live with a killer in the room*

In *Man's Search For Meaning*: Viktor Frankl, *Man's Search For Meaning,* first published in Austria in 1946.
Ruth's reading *The World I Fell Out Of*: Melanie Reid, *The World I Fell Out Of,* (4th Estate, 2019)

39 Jeffrey *and being part of something bigger than ourselves*

During what psychologist David Yaden refers to: David Bryce Yaden, Jonathan Haidt, Ralph W. Hood jr., David R. Vago, Andrew B. Newberg, 'The Varieties of Self-Transcendent Experiences,' *Review of General Psychology,* Vol 21, Issue 2, 2017.
alleviation of anxiety and depression: Stephen Ross, Anthony Bossis, Jeffrey Guss, Gabrielle Agin-Liebes, Tara Malone, Barry Cohen, Sarah E Mennenga, Alexander Belser, Krystallia Kalliontzi, James Babb, Zhe Su, Patricia Corby, Brian L Schmidt, 'Rapid and sustained symptom reduction

following psilocybin treatment for anxiety and depression in patients with life-threatening cancer: a randomized controlled trial,' *Journal of Psychopharmacology*, Vol 30, Issue 12, 2016.

However, a 2019 YouGov poll: retrieved from https://www.drugscience.org.uk/uk-psilocybin-support-yougov-poll/ on 5 October 2021.

parts of the broad, many-coloured river: Diana Athill, *Somewhere Towards the End,* (Granta, 2008), p83.

concentric circles of influence: Yalom, *Staring at the Sun,* p83.

ultimately we will come to nothing: *The Wiley Blackwell Handbook of Humanism,* introduction, p19.

In *The Power of Meaning*: Emily Esfahani Smith, *The Power of Meaning,* (Rider, 2017) pp143-148.

we ourselves are adding our grains of sand: Athill, *Somewhere Towards the End,* p180.

In his influential book *The Denial of Death*: Ernest Becker, *The Denial of Death* (Free Press, 1973) p151, p160.

Printed in Great Britain
by Amazon